Hormones and Atherosclerosis

Robert W. Stout, MD, FRCP
Professor of Geriatric Medicine
The Queen's University of Belfast

MTP PRESS LIMITED · LANCASTER · BOSTON · THE HAGUE
International Medical Publishers

Published in the UK and Europe by
MTP Press Limited
Falcon House
Lancaster, England

British Library Cataloguing in Publication Data

Stout, Robert W.
  Hormones and Atherosclerosis.
  1. Atherosclerosis   2. Hormones
  I. Title
  616.1'36071   RC692

  ISBN-13: 978-94-011-6266-1   e-ISBN-13: 978-94-011-6264-7
  DOI: 10.1007/978-94-011-6264-7

Published in the USA by
MTP Press
A division of Kluwer Boston Inc
190 Old Derby Street
Hingham, MA 02043, USA

Library of Congress Cataloging in Publication Data

Stout, Robert W.
  Hormones and atherosclerosis.
  Bibliography: p.
  Includes index.
  1. Atherosclerosis—Etiology.   2. Hormones—
Physiological effect.   I. Title. [DNLM:
1. Hormones.   2. Arteriosclerosis—Etiology.
WG 550 S925h]
RC692.S74 1982 616.1'3   82–12696

ISBN-13: 978-94-011-6266-1

Copyright © 1982 R. W. Stout
Softcover reprint of the hardcover 1st edition 1982

Hormones and
Atherosclerosis

Contents

Preface

As the acute infectious diseases recede in importance, and as the number of people surviving into middle and old age increases, the chronic 'degenerative' diseases assume greater importance as causes of death and disability. Of these diseases, atherosclerosis is by far the most prevalent and its consequences the most devastating. The search for the cause of atherosclerosis is consuming large amounts of resources of both money and research talent. As yet, the cause remains unknown.

Much of the research effort into atherosclerosis has been concerned with lipid metabolism. This is based on the knowledge that abnormalities of certain lipids and lipoproteins predispose to cardiovascular disease. Often the research has not been directly related to atherosclerosis and it is only recently that widespread attention has been paid to the artery. The development of methods of growing vascular endothelial and smooth muscle cells in culture has made possible detailed studies of the biology of the arterial wall.

There are a number of reasons why investigations of lipid metabolism alone will not identify the cause of atherosclerosis. First, only a minority of patients with cardiovascular disease have abnormal circulating lipids and lipoproteins. Second, there are three major predisposing factors for atherosclerosis which cannot be entirely explained by abnormal lipid metabolism – age, sex, and diabetes mellitus. Third, it is now clear that lipid is only one component of the atheromatous plaque, and incorporation of lipid may be a late feature of the development of the lesion.

Of the three predisposing factors mentioned above, sex and diabetes are associated with changes in hormone secretion. Other endocrine disorders, including abnormalities in thyroid hormone and growth hormone secretion, have also been associated with an increased frequency of cardiovascular disease. This book is an attempt to discuss the association of hormones and atherosclerosis.

The emphasis of the book is on atherosclerosis defined by the World Health Organization as 'a variable combination of changes of the intima of the arteries (as distinct from arterioles) consisting of the focal accumulation of lipids, complex carbohydrates, blood and blood products, fibrous tissue and calcium deposits and associated with medial changes'. Other types of vascular disease are not discussed, nor is thrombosis except where it closely relates to atherosclerosis. The emphasis is also on the major hormones and the clinical syndromes associated with their abnormalities. Other more recently discovered hormones, including the arachidonic acid metabolites associated with platelet function, are discussed in relation to the major hormones.

The literature on atherosclerosis is vast. Only references which are relevant to the topic discussed are included, although overlap with other topics is difficult to avoid and some pertinent reports may have been inadvertently omitted. I have concentrated on the recent literature and, with rare exceptions, have avoided citing abstracts. I hope that the reviews of the association of hormone secretion with atherosclerosis, and of the experimental evidence of hormone action on the arterial wall are comprehensive. The sections on lipid metabolism and other risk factors are inevitably more selective.

My interest in hormones and atherosclerosis was first stimulated 15 years ago by Professor John Vallence-Owen's suggestion that high insulin levels may predispose to vascular disease. With his active encouragement and support, I involved myself in experimental work in this topic in the Department of Medicine, The Queen's University of Belfast. The department was soon joined by Professor Keith Buchanan with whom I also enjoyed fruitful collaboration. In 1971 I was awarded an Eli Lilly Foreign Educational Fellowship by the Medical Research Council and spent 18 months at the University of Washington School of Medicine, Seattle, USA. There I had the good fortune to work in the Division of Gerontology and Metabolism which was headed by Dr Edwin Bierman, and which included Drs Daniel Porte, William Hazzard and John Brunzell. I also had the opportunity to work with Dr Russell Ross in the Department of Pathology. More recently Dr Hugh Taggart has investigated oestrogens and atherosclerosis in my own department. While I have quoted the published work of all these investigators, it is impossible to assess the impact on my thinking of the ideas formulated in many fruitful and enjoyable discussions. I acknowledge with gratitude the contributions of these friends and colleagues. I, of course, accept full responsibility for all that is written in this book.

Much of the basic work of this book was carried out while I was a visiting scientist at the University of Washington School of Medicine in spring 1981. I am grateful to the Wellcome Trust for financial assistance which made this visit possible. Libraries are of course essential for writers of a book of this type and I received great assistance from the Medical Library of the Queen's University of Belfast. I am particularly grateful to Dr Keith Lewis, assistant librarian, for considerable help. Mrs Melanie Hilary and Miss Andree Best typed the manuscript with great skill and patience. Lastly I thank my wife and family for their forbearance over many months when I shut myself in my study and was generally unsociable.

Acknowledgments

I am grateful to the following for permission to use copyright illustrations:

Figure 2.1 From *Diabetes, its Physiological and Biochemical Basis*, edited by J. Vallance-Owen, by kind permission of MTP Press, Lancaster.

Figure 4.1 From Chait, A., Bierman, E. L. and Albers, J. J. (1979). Low density lipoprotein receptor activity in fibroblasts cultured from diabetic donors. *Diabetes*, **28**, 914–18, by kind permission of Dr Alan Chait, and the American Diabetes Association Inc.

Figure 5.1 From Chait, A., Bierman, E. L. and Albers, J. J. (1978). Regulatory role of insulin in the degradation of low density lipoprotein by cultured human skin fibroblasts. *Biochim. Biophys. Acta*, **529**, 292–9, by kind permission of Dr Alan Chait and Elsevier Biomedical Press, Amsterdam.

Figure 6.1 From Stout, R. W. (1979). Diabetes and atheroscelerosis – the role of insulin. *Diabetologia*, **16**, 141–50, by kind permission of Springer-Verlag, Heidelberg.

Figure 7.2. From Stout, R. W., Buchanan, K. D. and Vallance-Owen, J. (1972). Arterial lipid metabolism in relation to blood glucose and plasma insulin in rats with streptozotocin-induced diabetes. *Diabetologia*, **8**, 398–401, by kind permission of Springer–Verlag.

Figure 7.3 From Stout, R. W., Bierman, E. L. and Ross, R. (1975). Effect of insulin on the proliferation of cultured primate arterial smooth muscle cells. *Circ. Res.*, **36**, 319–28, by kind permission of the American Heart Association.

Figure 15.1 From Chait, A., Bierman, E. L. and Albers, J. J. (1979). Regulatory role of triiodothyronine in the degradation of low density lipoprotein by cultured human skin fibroblasts. *J. Clin. Endocrinol. Metab.*, **48**, 887–9, by kind permission of Dr Alan Chait and the Editor in Chief, *Journal of Clinical Endocrinology and Metabolism*.

1
Introduction

Atherosclerosis is the major killing and disabling disease of adults in the developed world. It is a condition which occurs in everybody as age advances, and must be closely related to the biological process of ageing. On the other hand, atherosclerosis and its clinical complications may appear prematurely or in an unusually advanced degree in younger people. Often such people have certain inherited or acquired features in common. It is useful to consider atherosclerosis as a disease which is related to an intrinsic age-related process but which is modified by hereditary or environmental influences.

Atherosclerosis is difficult to diagnose except by complex and invasive radiological methods. These methods are unsuitable for epidemiological studies and would usually be considered unethical for pure research purposes. Thus, most of our knowledge of clinical atherosclerosis is based on studies of its complications. These include the various clinical manifestations of ischaemic heart disease, cerebrovascular disease and peripheral vascular disease, as well as death from cardiovascular disease and sudden death. The cause of fatal events may be confirmed by autopsy but this is not always performed. All these indirect methods of identifying atherosclerosis lack precision, particularly when more subjective characteristics, like angina pectoris, are used. They also have the disadvantage that only the late stages of the disease are being studied. Thus influences on the early development of the arterial lesions may no longer be operating when complete occlusion of a vessel occurs. The factors involved in the presentation of the late manifestations of atherosclerosis may be different from those operating on the arterial wall earlier in life.

Atherosclerosis starts in the late teens or early twenties. Advanced arterial disease has been found at autopsy in people accidentally killed at this age[1]. As it is only possible to examine a human atheromatous lesion once, the exact nature of the earliest lesions and the rate of their progression remain unknown. Because it is so difficult to study human atherosclerosis, animal models of the disease have been extensively used. The first animal model to gain widespread recognition was the cholesterol-fed rabbit, introduced by Anitschkow[2]. A large number of different animals fed high fat and cholesterol diets are now used. These models allow the rapid development of lipid-laden arterial lesions. However, it is not clear how closely they are related to the human disease, which develops very slowly, usually in people with normal plasma lipids.

Animal studies have placed a great deal of emphasis on circulating lipids and by extension, on dietary fat, and this has led to hypotheses linking dietary and circulating lipids to human atherosclerosis. This has resulted in a vast amount of research in human lipid metabolism. While this has led to a much greater understanding of the physiology and pathophysiology of human lipid metabolism and its disorders, it has not resulted in a corresponding increase in understanding of atherosclerosis. More recently, the technique of cell culture has been used in atherosclerosis research. This method allows cells of a defined type to be studied under carefully controlled conditions. Human arterial endothelial and smooth muscle cells have been successfully grown in culture. While the conditions of cultured cells can be rigorously controlled, there are many important differences between their culture environment and that *in vivo*. Thus, caution must be exercised in extrapolating the results of cell culture experiments to the whole organism.

Much of our knowledge of human atherosclerosis comes from epidemiological studies. These investigations have sought to identify special characteristics of people who develop the clinical complications of atherosclerosis. Prospective studies, where characteristics are identified in healthy people who are then followed for a period of time, provide the best evidence of an association between the characteristics and the disease. The study which has produced most information was carried out in Framingham, Massachusetts, USA[3]. The inhabitants of Framingham were initially examined in 1948 and have had biannual clinical and laboratory examinations since then. Initial characteristics which are associated with a high subsequent incidence of cardiovascular disease are called 'risk factors'. There have been many other smaller prospective studies of cardiovascular disease often specifically studying selected risk factors.

Risk factors identify the person who is at increased hazard of developing a disease. However, the exact relationship between the risk factor and the pathogenesis of the disease cannot be identified from epidemiological investigations. In particular, risk does not imply cause. The link between the risk factor and the pathological process may be indirect or the two may be linked by a third, perhaps unidentified, factor.

The Task Force on Arteriosclerosis of the National Heart and Lung Institute[4] carefully reviewed the published evidence and identified 12 risk factors (Table 1.1). Of these, the increased risk of atherosclerosis of the male sex, or the relative protection of the female sex, may be hormonally based, while diabetes, obesity and physical inactivity may be related and associated with changes in insulin secretion. Some types of hypertension are associated with abnormalities in the renin–angiotensin system. All of these will be discussed in later chapters of this book. Thyroid disorders will also be discussed, although the evidence is not sufficient to classify these as risk factors for cardiovascular disease. The evidence linking growth hormone and corticosteroids to atherosclerosis is even less impressive.

Table 1.1 Risk factors for atherosclerosis[4]

Age	Obesity
Male sex	Physical inactivity
Abnormal serum lipids	Genetic predisposition
Hypertension	Psychosocial stress
Cigarette smoking	Gout
Diabetes mellitus	Hardness of drinking water

The purpose of this book is to review the evidence linking changes in circulating hormone levels, of endogenous or exogenous origin, to atherosclerosis. For each hormone, an attempt is made to assess the strength of the link with atherosclerosis. Possible mechanisms, including effects on circulating lipids, are then discussed and finally experimental evidence of a direct effect of the hormone on the arterial wall is reviewed.

References

1. Enos, W. F., Holmes, R. J. and Beyer, J. (1953). Coronary disease among United States soldiers killed in action in Korea: preliminary report. *J. Am. Med. Assoc.*, **152**, 1090
2. Anitschkow, A. N. (1913). Uber Veranderungen der Kaninchen Aorta bei Experimenteller Cholesterinsteatose. *Beitr. Pathol. Anat. Allg. Pathol.*, **56**, 379
3. Kannel, W. B., Dawber, T. R., Friedman, G. D., Glennon, W. E. and McNamara, P. M. (1964). Risk factors in coronary heart disease. *Ann. Intern. Med.*, **61**, 888
4. National Heart and Lung Institute Task Force on Arteriosclerosis (1971). *Arteriosclerosis.* DHEW Publication No 72–219

2
The pathogenesis of atherosclerosis

THE ATHEROSCLEROTIC LESION

The normal artery is divided into three layers: the intima, media and adventitia. The adventitia consists of connective and adipose tissue, and its function is to relate the vessel to the surrounding tissues. It plays no part in the development of atherosclerosis and will not be considered further here. The media consists of smooth muscle cells, concentrically and longitudinally arranged. It is separated from the adventitia by the external elastic lamina and from the intima by the much more distinct fenestrated internal elastic lamina. The intima lines the luminal surface of the artery and consists of a thin layer of connective tissue containing, in the normal older artery, a small number of smooth muscle cells, and a single layer of epithelium-like endothelial cells. Atherosclerosis is a disease of the intima and inner media. The cells involved in the process are therefore endothelial and smooth muscle cells.

Endothelial cells have at least three functions[1] (Table 2.1). They act as a blood-compatible container allowing free flow of blood. To do this they must inhibit clotting within the vessel. This is accomplished both by the physical characteristics of the endothelial cells and by their synthesis and secretion of a potent platelet anti-aggregatory agent, prostacyclin. Second, endothelial cells act as a selectively permeable barrier allowing entry to the inner arterial wall of selected plasma constituents and excluding others. This is an active energy-requiring process. Third, endothelial cells synthesize, metabolize and secrete a number of substances, including prostacyclin, angiotensin-converting enzyme, clotting factor VIII and possibly, lipoprotein lipase. Endothelial cells may be grown in culture and human endothelial cells can be conveniently obtained from umbilical artery or vein[2,3]. Factors influencing the proliferation of endothelial cells are shown in Table 2.2.

Arterial smooth muscle cells also have a variety of functions[8] (Table 2.3). They provide the main structural support of the artery. By their contractile responses they regulate the size of the arterial lumen and hence blood flow

5

Table 2.1   Functions of endothelial cells

---

1. Blood-compatible container

2. Selective permeability barrier

3. Synthetic/metabolic/secretory tissue
   angiotensin-converting enzyme
   factor VIII
   plasminogen activator
   von Willebrand factor
   prostacyclin
   thromboxane
   fibronectin
   collagen (type IV)
   α-2-macroglobulin
   lipoprotein lipase
   hormone receptors
     adrenergic
     insulin
     oestrogen
     thrombin

4. Binding and internalization of lipoproteins

Table   2.2.   Factors   affecting   proliferation   of
                  endothelial cells

---

1. Serum[4]
2. Platelet factor (inhibits)[5]
3. Cyclic AMP (inhibits)[6]
4. Glucose (inhibits)[7]
5. Cell- and tissue-derived growth factors[4]

Table 2.3.   Functions of arterial smooth muscle cells

---

1. Structural support

2. Contractile responses

3. Synthetic/metabolic/secretory tissue
   actin
   myosin
   collagen
   elastin
   microfibrillar proteins
   proteoglycans
   lipids

4. Endocytosis

---

and blood pressure. They also have major synthetic functions and being the only cell type in the arterial media they are responsible for the synthesis of all constituents of the arterial wall. Smooth muscle cells are also capable of endocytosis of foreign material and lipoproteins. It has recently been suggested that arterial smooth muscle cells can exist in one of two forms – a contractile form or a synthetic form – and that proliferation is only possible in the synthetic form[8]. Under certain cultural conditions, smooth muscle cells can be observed to change from one form to another ('phenotypic modulation')[9]. Arterial smooth cells can be cultured from a number of species including man[10,11]. Factors influencing the proliferation of smooth muscle cells are shown in Table 2.4.

Table 2.4 Factors affecting the proliferation of arterial smooth muscle cells

1. Serum[10]
2. Hyperlipaemic serum and lipoproteins[12,13]
3. Diabetic serum[14]
4. Growth hormone[15]
5. Insulin[16]
6. Platelet factor[17]
7. Prostaglandins (inhibit)[18]
8. Cyclic AMP (inhibits)[6]

Atheromatous lesions are usually described as fatty streaks, mainly composed of foam cells; fibrous plaques, mainly composed of connective tissue; or complicated lesions, which contain calcium, lipid, connective tissue and often superimposed thrombosis. It is assumed, but cannot be proven, that the lesion progresses from a fatty streak to a fibrous plaque and hence to a complicated lesion. However, recent evidence obtained from studies of isoenzymes in arterial smooth muscle cells has confirmed the importance of the fatty streak in atherosclerosis[19]. The major constituents of the atheromatous lesion are smooth muscle cells, connective tissue and lipid.

THE DEVELOPMENT OF THE ATHEROSCLEROTIC LESION

In both humans and experimental animals, the earliest identifiable lesion is an accumulation of smooth muscle cells in the intima (Figure 2.1). These may result from replication of cells already in the intima or from proliferation and migration of medial smooth muscle cells. The smooth muscle cells then accumulate lipid, and extracellular lipid and connective tissue is laid down. The complicated lesion with calcification, haemorrhage, ulceration and superimposed thrombosis eventually develops. The lipid-filled cells of the lesion assume the characteristics of foam cells. At this stage it is difficult to identify the original cell type of the foam cell. They may be smooth muscle cells engorged with lipid or may originate from circulating monocyte macrophages[20].

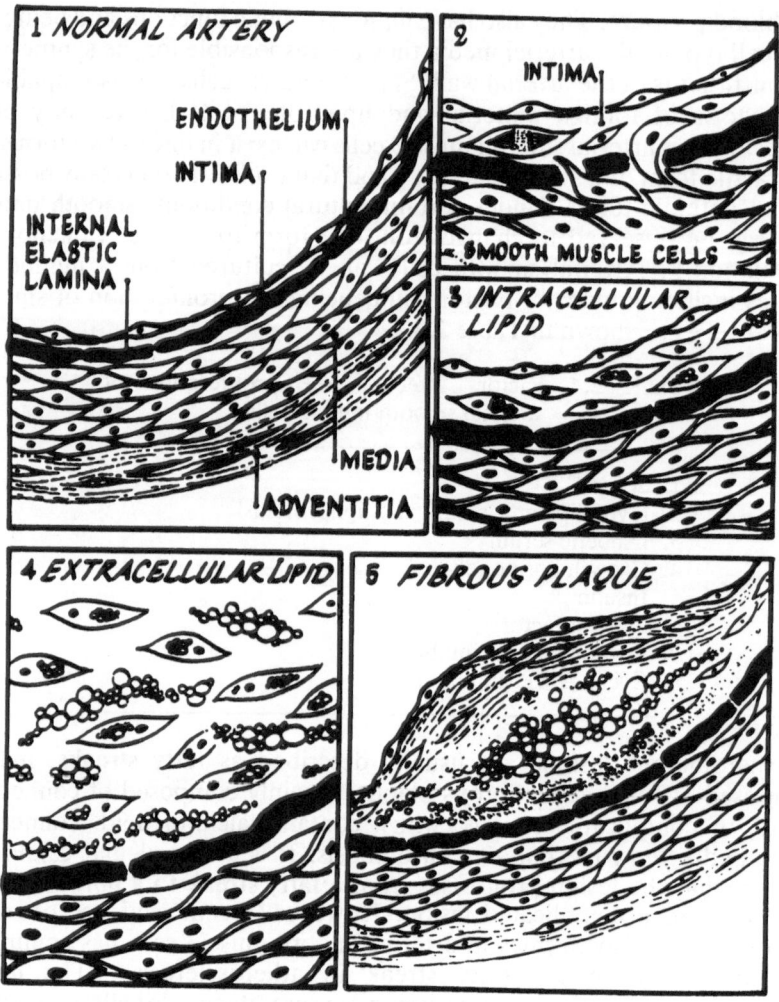

Figure 2.1 The development of atherosclerosis. The normal artery (1) consists of the intima, with a single layer of endothelial cells, the media composed of smooth muscle cells and the connective tissue adventitia. The earliest identifiable change is an increased number of smooth muscle cells in the intima (2). This is followed by intracellular (3) and extracellular (4) lipid accumulation and eventually the fibrous plaque (5) with connective tissue and calcification is formed

Theories on the pathogenesis of atherosclerosis have been proposed for many years[21]. These include the thrombogenic theory which suggested that the lesions develop from thrombus deposited on the arterial wall, the inflammatory theory which proposed that the lesion is an inflammatory response to degeneration of the arterial wall, the lipid theory which placed most importance on dietary and circulating lipids, and the insudation theory which suggested that an early change is accumulation of serous fluid derived from the blood. There are a number of more modern theories to explain the cellular basis of the development of the atheromatous lesion (Table 2.5). These theories are not mutually exclusive and while each has experimental support none can be regarded as conclusive.

Table 2.5 Theories of the cause of atherosclerosis

Response to injury	Lysosomal
Monoclonal	Clonal senescence

The *response to injury* theory[22] suggests that the earliest change is an injury or alteration to the endothelium. This allows the entry into the inner parts of the arterial wall of plasma constituents and these act on the artery to produce the lesion. Removal of endothelium exposes the subendothelial collagen to which platelets rapidly adhere. Adhesion and aggregation of platelets is followed by release of the contents of the platelet granules. These include a potent mitogen, the platelet-derived growth factor[17] which initiates proliferation of smooth muscle cells. Other plasma constituents including insulin and lipoproteins act in a co-ordinated fashion to permit multiple rounds of cell division after exposure of the cells to platelet factor[8]. The smooth muscle cells then take up lipoproteins and synthesize connective tissue. The early changes are considered to be a repair process following injury to the endothelium and under certain conditions the changes regress and the integrity of the arterial wall is restored. In other circumstances the process continues to the formation of the advanced lesion.

Evidence for the response to injury theory comes from studies on experimental animals. Mechanical removal of the endothelium with balloon catheters results in smooth muscle cell proliferation[23]. If the animals are on a high-fat diet lesions develop, while on a normal diet the smooth muscle cell proliferation regresses. If platelet activity is suppressed pharmacologically[24] or is congenitally deficient[25] lesions do not occur. Cell culture studies of arterial smooth muscle cells have identified growth factors including platelet factor[17], insulin[16] and lipoproteins[13].

The *monoclonal* theory[26] suggests that the proliferating smooth muscle cells originate from a single cell, i.e. they are monoclonal in origin. In this respect the atheromatous lesion resembles a benign smooth muscle cell tumour. Evidence for the monoclonal theory has come from studies of glucose-6-phosphate dehydrogenase (G-6-PD) isoenzymes in ather-omatous plaques of women who are heterozygous for G-6-PD deficiency[27]. The pattern of isoenzymes in the plaques is consistent with a monoclonal origin of the cells. The techniques of isoenzyme identification have also been used to follow the progress of atheromatous lesions[19]. The monoclonal theory suggests that only selected smooth muscle cells proliferate in response to stimulation by growth factors. These cells may have a genetic predisposition or may have undergone a mutation.

The *lysosomal* theory[28] suggests that a fault in lysosome activity results in accumulation of lipid within the cells of the lesion. Lysosomes are intracellular organelles which are concerned with catabolism. It is suggested that the accumulation of intracellular lipid results from a defect in lysosomal activity and hence impaired catabolism of intracellular particles. Cell fractionation studies in atheromatous lesions provide evidence for lysosomal dysfunction in atherosclerosis.

The *clonal senescence* theory[29] relates atherosclerosis to ageing. It is based not on growth factors, but on factors which inhibit cell replication. The ultimate size of any organ results from finely regulated cell growth. This is under the control of both growth-promoting factors and factors, called chalones, which inhibit cell growth. The clonal senescence theory suggests that arterial smooth muscle cell proliferation results from the selective age-related decline of cells which produce chalones resulting in uninhibited proliferation of the remaining smooth muscle cells.

If the response to injury theory is regarded as the basic mechanism of atherogenesis then the monoclonal, lysosomal and clonal senescence theories can all be accommodated within it. It is likely that some of these mechanisms operate in some cases of atherosclerosis and others, including some not yet identified, operate in others. The complicated atheromatous lesion can be regarded as the end-stage of a variety of different pathophysiological processes. Evidence on the nature of the initial process is by that stage obliterated.

LIPID METABOLISM

The regulation of lipid and lipoprotein metabolism has been the subject of a number of recent comprehensive reviews[30–32] and only a brief summary is given here.

The major lipids in the human circulation are triglyceride, cholesterol and cholesterol esters, phospholipids, and fatty acids. These lipids are insoluble in water and therefore means exist to allow them to circulate in an aqueous medium. Free fatty acids circulate in association with plasma albumin, a complex which is not designated a lipoprotein. Triglyceride, cholesterol and phospholipids circulate in combination with specific peptides, apolipoproteins or apoproteins, forming a family of particles known as lipoproteins.

Lipoproteins may be separated by their physical properties, particularly electrical charge and density. The common laboratory methods used for separating lipoproteins are electrophoresis and ultracentrifugation. Electrophoresis is essentially a qualitative method and is only of importance now because one of the nomenclatures for lipoproteins is based on electrophoretic mobility. The commonest method of separating lipoproteins for clinical studies is based on their density and uses a single separation by ultracentrifugation combined with precipitation. Lipoproteins may be separated more accurately by sequential ultracentrifugation and by analytical ultracentrifugation.

Using these methods of separation four main classes of lipoproteins can be distinguished. In increasing order of density these are chylomicrons, very low-density lipoproteins (VLDL), low-density lipoproteins (LDL) and high-density lipoproteins (HDL). When electrophoresis is used the nomenclature of lipoproteins is as follows: VLDL are known as pre-beta-lipoproteins, LDL as beta-lipoproteins and HDL as alpha-lipoproteins. In this discussion the density nomenclature will be used. These classes represent families of lipoproteins and some other lipoproteins are also identified under certain circumstances. These include the intermediate-density lipoproteins, intermediate between the VLDL and the LDL, and subclasses of the HDL family.

The composition and physical properties of the major lipoproteins are shown in Table 2.6. Chylomicrons are formed in the intestinal mucosa and are the means of carrying dietary or exogenous triglyceride from the gut to the circulation and hence to the liver and adipose tissue. Chylomicrons are found in the circulation after a fatty meal but are not normally present after an overnight fast. They float on top of plasma, forming a creamy layer in plasma which has been stored at 4 °C overnight, and remain at the origin in standard electrophoretic techniques. VLDL transport endogenously synthesized triglyceride. VLDL are synthesized in the liver but some VLDL results from the catabolism of chylomicrons with removal of triglyceride by the enzyme lipoprotein lipase. Chylomicrons and VLDL are the major triglyceride-carrying lipoproteins of the plasma.

LDL are formed as a result of the catabolism of VLDL. After lipolysis of VLDL triglyceride mediated by lipoprotein lipase an intermediate-density lipoprotein (IDL) formed. This is present only transiently in the circulation under normal conditions. The IDL is further metabolized by the liver and appears as LDL. The smallest lipoprotein is the HDL. Its origin is unknown but it may be a product of the catabolism of VLDL with further modification under the influence of the enzyme, lecithin-cholesterol acyl transferase (LCAT).

The concentration of triglyceride in the circulation is a balance between synthesis and removal. Circulating triglyceride has two sources: the diet and endogenous synthesis in the liver. Synthesis of triglyceride is governed by the availability of free fatty acid and glucose substrate to the liver, and is influenced by insulin. Removal of triglyceride from the circulation depends on lipoprotein lipase, which is also influenced by insulin. The fatty acids resulting from lipolysis of plasma triglyceride pass into adipose tissue to be re-esterified as storage triglyceride, while the glycerol returns to the liver for further metabolism. Triglyceride synthesis and removal are also under genetic influence. Some familial hypertriglyceridaemias result from over-production of triglyceride by the liver, while others result from genetically determined deficiency in lipoprotein lipase.

The major lipid of the atheromatous lesion is cholesterol, most of which is in the esterified form. In the circulation the main cholesterol-carrying lipoprotein is LDL, but some cholesterol is also carried by VLDL and by HDL which transport cholesterol away from cells. LDL interact with specific cell membrane receptors which are situated in coated pits on the surface of extrahepatic cells[32]. The LDL receptor complex is then

Table 2.6 Composition and physical properties of lipoproteins

	Protein	Triglyceride	Cholesterol	Phospholipid	Major Apoproteins	S_f	Density	Mobility
			%					
Chylomicrons	2	85	4	9	A-I, A-II, B	400	0.95	Origin
VLDL	10	50	15	18	C-I, C-II, C-III	20–400	0.95–1.006	pre-β
LDL	23	10	45	20	B, C-I, C-II	0.20	1.006–1.063	β
HDL	55	4	17	24	C-III, E	$F_{1.20}$0–9	1.063–1.21	α

internalized by invagination of the coated pits which form endocytic vesicles carrying the LDL to the lysosomes. The protein component (apoprotein) of the lipoprotein is degraded and extruded from the cell and the cholesterol ester is hydrolysed. The released cholesterol has three effects in the cell:

(1) inhibition of the enzyme 3-hydroxy-3-methylglutaryl coenzyme A reductase (HMG-CoA reductase) the rate-limiting enzyme in the cholesterol synthetic pathway resulting in decreased intracellular cholesterol synthesis;
(2) stimulation of intracellular cholesterol esterification;
(3) suppression of synthesis of LDL receptors on the cell membrane.

Thus interaction of LDL with its receptor results in degradation of the lipoprotein, suppression of intracellular cholesterol synthesis and enhancement of intracellular cholesterol esterification. In experimental animals it has been found the LDL is catabolized in the absence of a functioning liver, suggesting that LDL is broken down in peripheral tissues.

The other lipoproteins also interact with cell membrane receptors. The macromolecular complexes that originate from partial removal of triglyceride from VLDL (IDL) or chylomicrons (remnants) leaving relatively cholesterol-rich particles, are avidly taken up by cellular receptor mechanisms, including the LDL receptor[33,34]. HDL competes with LDL for its receptor and hence high ratios of HDL to LDL tend to reduce LDL uptake[35]. While receptor-mediated uptake in extrahepatic cells, particularly fibroblasts, is an important physiological mechanism for the removal of LDL from the circulation, large amounts of LDL can also be taken up by scavenger cells, particularly monocyte-macrophages, by non-receptor mechanisms[36]. Engorgement of lipid results in the formation of foam cells.

The LDL receptor is a major regulating mechanism in the transport and metabolism of the lipoprotein. Receptor activity can be modified by genetic diseases (familial hypercholesterolaemia) and by hormones (Table 2.7). LDL receptor activity is likely to be an important mechanism in both lipid metabolism and atherosclerosis.

Table 2.7 Factors which increase (↑) or decrease (↓) extrahepatic LDL receptors

Active growth (↑)[32]
Quiescent growth (↓)[32]
Excess cellular cholesterol (↓)[32]
Cholesterol deprivation (↑)[32]
Insulin (↑)[37]
Thyroxin (↑)[38]
Platelet-derived growth factor (↑)[39]
Cyclic AMP (↓)[40]

References

1. Gimbrone, M. A. Jr. (1979). Endothelial dysfunction and the pathogenesis of atherosclerosis. In Gotto, A. M., Smith, L. C. and Allen, B. (eds.) *Atherosclerosis*. Vol. 5, pp. 415–26. (New York: Springer-Verlag)
2. Jaffe, E. A., Nachman, R. L., Becker, C. G. and Minick, C. R. (1973). Culture of human endothelial cells derived from umbilical veins. Identification by morphologic and immunologic criteria. *J. Clin. Invest.*, **52**, 2745
3. Gimbrone, M. A. Jr, Cotran, R. S. and Folkman, J. (1974). Human vascular endothelial cells in culture. *J. Cell. Biol.*, **60**, 673
4. Schwartz, S. M., Gajdusek, C. M. and Selden, S. C. III. (1981). Vascular wall growth control: the role of the endothelium. *Arteriosclerosis*, **1**, 107
5. Taggart, H. and Stout, R. W. (1980). Control of DNA synthesis in cultured vascular endothelial and smooth muscle cells – response to serum, platelet-deficient serum, lipid-free serum, insulin and oestrogens. *Atherosclerosis*, **37**, 549
6. Stout, R. W. (1982). Cyclic AMP: a potent inhibitor of DNA synthesis in cultured arterial endothelial and smooth muscle cells. *Diabetologia*, **22**, 51
7. Stout, R. W. (1982). Glucose inhibits DNA synthesis in cultured human endothelial cells. *Diabetologia*. (In press)
8. Chamley-Campbell, J., Campbell, G. R. and Ross, R. (1979). The smooth muscle cell in culture. *Physiol. Rev.*, **59**, 1
9. Chamley-Campbell, J. H. and Campbell, G. R. (1981). What controls smooth muscle phenotype? *Atherosclerosis*, **40**, 347
10. Ross, R. (1971). The smooth muscle cell. II. Growth of smooth muscle in culture and formation of elastic fibres. *J. Cell Biol.*, **50**, 172
11. Bierman, E. L. and Albers, J. J. (1975). Lipoprotein uptake by cultured human arterial smooth muscle cells. *Biochim. Biophys. Acta*, **388**, 198
12. Fischer-Dzoga, K., Fraser, R. and Wissler, R. W. (1976). Stimulation of proliferation in stationary primary cultures of monkey and rabbit aortic smooth muscle cells. I. Effects of lipoprotein fractions of hyperlipemic serum and lymph. *Exp. Mol. Pathol.*, **24**, 346
13. Ross, R. and Glomset, J. A. (1973). Atherosclerosis and the arterial smooth muscle cell. *Science*, **180**, 1332
14. Ledet, T. (1976). Growth of rabbit aortic smooth muscle cells in serum from patients with juvenile diabetes. *Acta Pathol. Microbiol. Scand., Sect. A*, **84**, 508
15. Ledet, T. (1977). Growth hormone antiserum suppresses the growth effect of diabetic serum. *Diabetes*, **26**, 798
16. Stout, R. W., Bierman, E. L. and Ross, R. (1975). Effect of insulin on the proliferation of cultured primate arterial smooth muscle cells. *Circ. Res.*, **36**, 319
17. Ross, R. and Vogel, A. (1978). The platelet-derived growth factor. *Cell*, **14**, 203
18. Huttner, J. J., Gwebu, E. T., Panganamala, R. V., Milo, G. E. and Cornwell, D.G. (1977). Fatty acids and their prostaglandin derivatives: inhibitors of proliferation in aortic smooth muscle cells. *Science*, **197**, 289
19. Pearson, T. A., Dillman, J. M., Solez, K. and Heptinstall, R. H. (1980). Evidence for two populations of fatty streaks with different roles in the atherogenic process. *Lancet*, **2**, 496
20. Gerrity, R. G. (1981). The role of the monocyte in atherogenesis. *Am. J. Pathol.*, **103**, 181
21. Haust, M. D. and More, R. H. (1972). Development of modern theories on the pathogenesis of atherosclerosis. In Wissler, R. W. and Geer, J. C. (eds.). *The Pathogenesis of Atherosclerosis*, pp. 1–19. (Baltimore: Williams & Wilkins)
22. Ross, R. and Glomset, J. A. (1976). The pathogenesis of atherosclerosis. *N. Engl. J. Med.*, **295**, 369, 420
23. Spaet, T. H., Stemerman, M. B., Veith, F. J. and Lejnieks, I. (1975). Intimal injury and regrowth in the rabbit aorta. Medial smooth muscle cells as a source of neointima. *Circ. Res.*, **36**, 58
24. Friedman, R. J., Stemerman, M. B., Wenz, B. *et al.* (1977). The effect of thrombocytopenia on experimental arteriosclerotic lesion formation in rabbits. Smooth muscle cell proliferation and re-endothelialization. *J. Clin. Invest.*, **60**, 1191
25. Fuster, V., Bowie, E. J. W., Lewis, J. C., Fass, D. N., Owen, C. A. Jr and Brown, A. L.

(1978). Resistance to arteriosclerosis in pigs with von Willebrand's disease. Spontaneous and high cholesterol diet-induced arteriosclerosis. *J. Clin. Invest.*, **61**, 722

26. Benditt, E. P. and Benditt, J. M. (1973). Evidence for a monoclonal origin of human atherosclerotic plaques. *Proc. Natl. Acad. Sci., USA*, **70**, 1753
27. Pearson, T. A., Dillman, J. M., Solez, K. and Heptinstall, R. H. (1978). Clonal markers in the study of the origin and growth of human atherosclerotic lesions. *Circ. Res.*, **43**, 10
28. Wolinsky, H. (1980). A proposal linking clearance of circulating lipoproteins to tissue metabolic activity as a basis for understanding atherogenesis. *Circ. Res.*, **47**, 301
29. Martin, G. M. and Sprague, C. A. (1973). Symposium on *in vitro* studies related to atherogenesis life histories of hyperplastoid cell lines from aorta and skin. *Exp. Mol. Pathol.*, **18**, 125
30. Lewis, B. (1976). The hyperlipidemias. Clinical and laboratory practice. (Oxford: Blackwell)
31. Brunzell, J. D., Chait, A. and Bierman, E. L. (1978). Pathophysiology of lipoprotein transport. *Metabolism*, **27**, 1109
32. Brown, M. S., Kovanen, P. T. and Goldstein, J. L. (1981). Regulation of plasma cholesterol by lipoprotein receptors. *Science*, **212**, 628
33. Beirman, E. L., Eisenberg, S., Stein, O. and Stein, Y. (1973). Very low density lipoprotein 'remnant' particles: uptake by aortic smooth muscle cells in culture. *Biochim. Biophys. Acta*, **329**, 163
34. Floren, C.-H., Albers, J. J. and Bierman, E. L. (1981). Uptake of chylomicron remnants causes cholesterol accumulation in cultured human arterial smooth muscle cells. *Biochim. Biophys. Acta*, **663**, 336
35. Carew, T. E., Koschinsky, T., Hayes, S. B. and Steinberg, D. (1976). A mechanism by which high density lipoproteins may slow the atherogenetic process. *Lancet*, **1**, 1315
36. Goldstein, J. L., Ho, Y. K., Basu, S.K. and Brown, M. S. (1979). Binding site on macrophages that mediates uptake and degradation of acetylated low density lipoprotein, producing massive cholesterol deposition. *Proc. Natl. Acad. Sci., USA*, **76**, 333
37. Chait, A., Bierman, E. L. and Albers, J. J. (1978). Regulatory role of insulin in the degradation of low density lipoprotein by cultured human skin fibroblasts. *Biochim. Biophys. Acta*, **529**, 292
38. Chait, A., Bierman, E. L. and Albers, J. J. (1979). Regulatory role of triiodothyronine in the degradation of low density lipoprotein by cultured human skin fibroblasts. *J. Clin. Endocrinol. Metab.*, **48**, 887
39. Chait, A., Ross, R., Albers, J. J. and Bierman, E. L. (1980). Platelet-derived growth factor stimulates activity of low density lipoprotein receptors. *Proc. Natl. Acad. Sci., USA*, **77**, 4084
40. Stout, R. W. and Bierman, E. L. (1982). Dibutyryl cyclic AMP inhibits LDL binding in cultured fibroblasts and arterial smooth muscle cells. Atherosclerosis (in press)

DIABETES MELLITUS

3
Diabetes mellitus and atherosclerosis

Until insulin became available the association of diabetes with atherosclerosis was virtually unknown. There are a number of reasons for this. Survival of diabetics before insulin was introduced was short, and death was frequently due to ketoacidosis (Table 3.1). The milder type of diabetes now known as non-insulin-dependent diabetes mellitus (NIDDM) was not widely recognized and the clinical diagnosis of coronary heart disease was uncommon. Nevertheless, there were a few reports in the late nineteenth century and the first two decades of the twentieth century in which atherosclerosis and disorders of lipid metabolism were noted in diabetics (quoted by West 1978[2]). Since the 1920s a large number of studies have identified a high frequency of cardiovascular disease in diabetes. Despite modern treatment the expectation of life in diabetics is still considerably shorter than that of non-diabetics (Table 3.2) but the commonest cause of death in diabetics is now atherosclerotic cardiovascular disease. Diabetes and atherosclerosis has been the subject of a number of reviews by the author and colleagues[3,4] as well as by others[2].

A clear distinction must be drawn between two types of vascular lesion which occur in diabetics. Disease of the small vessels, particularly the capillaries (microangiopathy), is common in diabetics and particularly

Table 3.1 Causes of death in 27 966 diabetics (percentages)[1]

	1897–1922	1922–36	1937–49	1950–59	1960–68
Diabetic coma	52.6	8.3	2.3	1.0	1.0
Arteriosclerotic	20.9	54.0	68.0	75.8	75.0
Cardiac	8.0	29.8	44.2	50.6	53.8
Coronary and angina	1.8	12.4	24.8	34.3	41.9
Infections	10.1	13.6	8.2	5.2	5.6
Cancer	2.7	8.7	9.4	10.6	11.6

Table 3.2 Expectation of life in diabetics and non-diabetics according to age of onset of diabetes[79]

Age of onset of diabetes	Mortality ratio (%)	Expectation of life (years)	
		Diabetics	Non-diabetics
Under 15	1127	32	59
15–19	926	33	56
20–29	443	33	49
30–39	344	28	39
40–49	301	20	30
50–59	213	17	23
60–70	234	11	16

affects the retina and the renal glomerulus. This type of disease is thought to be specific to diabetes and is unrelated to the macroangiopathy. The large vessel disease that occurs in diabetics is caused by atherosclerosis and this does not differ in morphologic appearance or in biochemical composition from atherosclerosis in non-diabetics[5].

Much of the epidemiological and clinical data associating diabetes with atherosclerosis has used as evidence of atherosclerosis such clinical syndromes as myocardial infarction, angina pectoris, peripheral vascular disease and cerebrovascular disease. Sudden death and congestive cardiac failure have also been used as end-points. However, the latter categories are less clearly linked to atherosclerosis in the coronary circulation than the former categories. There is now accumulating evidence that diabetics are predisposed to disease of the left ventricular myocardium that is not only due to coronary atherosclerosis but appears to be also a result of metabolic abnormalities in the heart muscle itself[4]. This in some cases may be related to small-vessel disease in the myocardium but in other cases it can be reversed by correction of the metabolic abnormalities. It is clear therefore that not all heart disease in diabetics is due to atherosclerosis and the results of studies using congestive cardiac failure or death as end-points must be interpreted with caution as it is likely that a mixture of heart disease has been studied.

The earlier studies of atherosclerosis in diabetes did not use current classifications of diabetes mellitus. Diabetes in adults can be classified into two large categories[6]. A minority of diabetics have insulin-dependent diabetes mellitus (IDDM) which usually develops in adolescence or early adult life, is dependent on injected insulin to prevent the development of ketoacidosis, and is associated with specific HLA types and the presence of circulating anti-islet cell antibodies. The other category of diabetes is NIDDM. This usually develops in middle age and these diabetics are usually overweight, are not prone to develop ketoacidosis and do not have the immunological features found in IDDM. The relationship of atherosclerosis to the different types of diabetes has not been studied.

AUTOPSY STUDIES

In 1924, soon after the introduction of treatment of diabetes with insulin, Fitz and Murphy[7] reported that 24% of 64 fatal cases of diabetes had cardiovascular disease while Warren and Root in 1925[8] reported a high prevalence of coronary sclerosis in diabetes. Since 1930 many autopsy studies have been carried out and the results of a number of these are summarized in Table 3.3. The largest autopsy study of diabetes and atherosclerosis was the International Atherosclerosis Project[20] in which specimens from a number of different countries were examined. The coronary arteries and abdominal aortae of the diabetics showed more atherosclerosis than those of non-diabetics regardless of sex, age, race or geographic location.

Table 3.3 Autopsy ischaemic heart disease in diabetics and non-diabetics (percentages)

Study	Diabetic	Non-diabetic
Blottner (1930)[9]	45	21
Root and Sharkey (1930)[10]	32	6
Nathanson (1932)[11]	53	8
Root et al. (1939)[12]	32	6
Robbins and Tucker (1944)[13]	11	4
	(occlusion only)	
Stearns et al. (1947)[14]	64	23
Editorial (1948)[15]	67	—
Clawson and Bell (1949)[16]	20	9
Feldman and Feldman (1954)[17]	44	20
Liebow et al. (1955)[18]	42	—
Breithaupt and Leckie (1961)[19]	61	42

There have been a few reports which disagree with the finding of a high frequency of atherosclerosis in diabetics. For example, the Oxford necropsy survey did not find a significant increase in the degree of atherosclerosis in diabetics compared to normals[21]. However, the number of diabetics in this study was very small and excessive coronary atheroma was found in diabetics who had coronary thrombosis.

Three recent studies have applied modern techniques to the autopsy study of atherosclerosis in diabetics. In the Mayo Clinic the hearts of diabetics were examined and the degree of cross-sectional area narrowing by atherosclerotic plaques of each of the four major epicardial arteries was measured[22]. The patients had all attended the diabetes clinic but they had a mixture of insulin-dependent and non-insulin-dependent diabetes. The diabetics were grouped into those with or without clinical evidence of coronary heart disease, and the control group consisted of age- and sex-matched subjects who had had fatal coronary events but not diabetes. There were no controls who had neither diabetes nor coronary heart disease. The study disclosed similar degrees of severe narrowing by atherosclerotic plaques in the main coronary arteries in diabetic patients with or without clinical evidence of coronary heart disease and in non-diabetics with fatal coronary heart disease. There was no evidence of increased involvement of distal or smaller coronary arteries in the diabetics compared to the controls. The degree of coronary artery narrowing was not related to the age of onset, the duration of diabetes, the treatment used, or the random blood sugar levels. The most frequent fatal coronary event in the diabetics was acute myocardial infarction followed by 'sudden coronary death' and congestive cardiac failure. The frequency of these three types of fatal cardiac disease was not altered by the patient's age at onset of diabetes or by the duration of the diabetes. A major difference between the diabetics and the non-diabetics was found on examination of the left main coronary artery – there was a significantly higher frequency of severe narrowing of the left main coronary artery in the diabetics. In addition, healed transmural ventricular scars occurred more frequently in the diabetics than in the non-diabetic controls. Because of the multiple groups studied and the absence of a control group without either diabetes or coronary artery disease, the interpretation of this study is somewhat difficult. Nevertheless, it is clear that atherosclerosis is not related to the duration or severity of diabetes as currently assessed but that disease of the most significant coronary artery occurs more frequently in diabetics than in non-diabetics. Another autopsy study published at the same time reported the results of an examination of the hearts of 185 patients who had clinically established diabetes of adult onset but of mixed type[23]. The coronary arteries were examined by standardized coronary arteriographic techniques and the severity of diabetes was assessed by a review of the medical records. Once again there was no significant association between the degree of coronary artery atherosclerosis and the duration or severity of diabetes. Similarly there was no significant correlation between the severity of diabetes and atherosclerosis in other vessels throughout the body. The type of treatment of diabetes was not related to the degree of coronary atherosclerosis. However, when the diabetic group was compared with an age- and sex-matched control group without diabetes, the diabetics had significantly more coronary atherosclerosis. The number of diseased coronary arteries, the number of myocardial infarctions, the diffuseness of the coronary atherosclerosis and the presence of coronary arterial collatoral channels were all significantly greater in the diabetics than in the non-diabetics. While these results suggest that diabetics have more extensive atherosclerosis than non-diabetics, they also suggest that the progress of coronary atherosclerosis in diabetes of adult onset is independent of the progress of the diabetes itself.

While it is often stated that atherosclerosis occurs at a younger age in diabetics than non-diabetics, there is little good evidence to support this. However, an autopsy study of young diabetics has been reported[24]. Nine patients, average age 29 years, with insulin-dependent diabetes (average

age at onset 9 years) were compared with nine age-matched control subjects. The diabetics had significantly more extramural coronary narrowing than the controls and both the degree of narrowing and the extent of coronary arterial involvement were greater in the diabetics. In the diabetics 47% of the entire length of the coronary arteries was narrowed more than 50%, compared with only 1% of the length of the non-diabetic controls. Again there was no evidence of a significant abnormality in the small coronary vessels. Atherosclerosis was not present to a severe degree in all the diabetics. In two diabetics little coronary artery narrowing was found, and it was suggested that this was related to the infrequent occurrence of ketoacidosis in these subjects.

Thus with the notable exception of the Oxford study there is widespread agreement that atherosclerosis is more severe at all ages and occurs at a younger age in diabetics than in non-diabetics. Coronary atherosclerosis is not an inevitable accompaniment of diabetes and, since atherosclerosis is so common in non-diabetics, diabetes must have a facilitative rather than a causative role in the pathogenesis of the condition. Atherosclerosis in diabetes is not related to the duration of the diabetes, the age of onset of the disease, the blood glucose levels or the type of treatment. The results of the autopsy studies are particularly significant as clinical and epidemiological studies usually rely on less direct methods of diagnosis of atherosclerosis.

GLUCOSE TOLERANCE IN PATIENTS WITH ISCHAEMIC VASCULAR DISEASE

It has been known for many years that a large proportion of patients with ischaemic vascular disease have glycosuria or glucose intolerance. For example, Levine in 1922[25] found 7% of a group of patients with angina pectoris had diabetes and in 1929 he reported[28] a frequency of glycosuria of 24% in patients with coronary thrombosis. As the incidence of diabetes in adult life is around 2% these figures indicate an overrepresentation of abnormal glucose regulation in subjects with ischaemic heart disease. Levine pointed out that 'the relationship between diabetes and coronary disease needs more particular emphasis'. Some reports of diabetes and ischaemic vascular disease are summarized in Table 3.4.

The definitions of diabetes vary in the different studies. Nevertheless, the definitions are consistent in those with atherosclerosis and those without, and hence for comparative purposes the high incidence of diabetes in ischaemic vascular disease can be accepted. Other relevant figures include a frequency of glucose intolerance of 95% in patients who had amputations for ischaemic disease[39], a large proportion of diabetics among apparently healthy men with 'non-specific' T-wave abnormalities on their electrocardiograms[40], and a higher mortality, less pain, and a higher incidence of previous cardiac disease in diabetics with myocardial infarction[37].

More recently attention has been directed to abnormalities of carbohydrate metabolism which do not meet the criteria for diabetes in

Table 3.4 Frequency of diabetes (percentages) in clinical ischaemic vascular disease and in general hospital admissions

(a) Clinical ischaemic vascular disease	%
Levine (1922)[25]	7
Nathanson (1925)[26]	25
Kahn (1926)[27]	13
Levine (1929)[28]	24
Connor and Holt (1930)[29]	10
Master *et al.* (1939)[30]	11
Aarseth (1953)[31]	11
Bartels and Rullo (1958)[32].	20
Sievers *et al.* (1961)[33]	10
Fabrykant and Gelfand (1964)[34]	10
Conrad (1967)[35]	12
Datey and Nanda (1967)[36]	15
Bailey and Beavan (1968)[37]	8
(b) General admissions to hospital	
Conrad (1967)[35]	2
Bailey and Beavan (1968)[37]	4
Reid *et al.* (1974)[38]	1
	(males age 40–64)

patients with ischaemic vascular disease. Glucose tolerance has been determined by oral and intravenous methods and a variety of techniques have been used with loads of glucose ranging from 15 to 100 g. The findings of a number of these studies are summarized in Table 3.5. In the table the heading 'abnormal' denotes collectively the results described as diabetic, abnormal, pathological and borderline by different authors. The frequency of abnormal glucose tolerance tests in patients with ischaemic vascular disease is consistently high and results obtained with oral and intravenous glucose are almost identical. In all the studies the majority of patients with ischaemic vascular disease had abnormal glucose tolerance tests. The consistency of the results is particularly striking as the methods as well as the selection of the study subjects varied considerably.

A review of both the German and English literature on glucose tolerance in ischaemic vascular disease has found 61% of 590 oral glucose tolerance tests and 55% of 537 intravenous tolerance tests to be abnormal in patients with ischaemic vascular disease[50]. Intravenous glucose tolerance was the same in a homogeneous sample of survivors of a first attack of myocardial infarction as in patients who had one or more infarctions, angina pectoris or intermittent claudication with widely differing duration of ischaemic vascular disease. Age, obesity, diabetic heredity, sex and hypertension did not exert any influence on glucose tolerance in ischaemic vascular disease. Only two studies used age-matched controls but in the other studies the ages of the two groups were similar. While glucose intolerance may occur in

Table 3.5 Ischaemic vascular disease – oral glucose tolerance and intravenous glucose tolerance

Study	No. of cases	Abnormal glucose tolerance %
(a) Oral glucose tolerance		
Raab and Rabinowitz (1936)[41]	21	71
Goldberger et al. (1945)[42]	14	71
Waddell and Field (1960)[43]	47	85
Sowton (1962)[44]	30	73
Reaven et al. (1963)[45]	41	41
Fabrykant and Gelfand (1964)[34]	42	64
Reissell et al. (1964)[46]	10	70
Cohen and Shafrir (1965)[47]	43	77
Datey and Nanda (1967)[36]	145	67
Jakobson et al. (1968)[48]	41	54
TOTAL	434	64
(b) Intravenous glucose tolerance		
Wahlberg (1966)[49]	530	56

the acute phase of myocardial infarction as in other acute illnesses, certain facts suggest that acute stress is not the explanation for the findings of the studies quoted. Thus glucose tolerance tests repeated several weeks after the acute ischaemic episode showed similar results to the initial tests[50]. A mortality rate of 27% occurred in patients with abnormal glucose tolerance compared to 12% in patients with normal glucose tolerance[49]. This is comparable to the poor prognosis of ischaemic heart disease in manifest diabetes. Six months after the acute episode the majority of abnormal glucose tolerance tests remained abnormal[50].

Two studies of glucose tolerance in patients with angiographically proven coronary artery disease without myocardial infarction have been reported[51-54]. In each case 66% of subjects with coronary atheroma had abnormal glucose tolerance compared with 18–25% of those with normal arteries. Nearly 60% of patients with arterial disease had abnormal lipoproteins compared to 9% controls and over 50% had abnormalities in serum cholesterol and triglyceride levels. Other evidence that it is arterial disease itself, rather than cardiac damage, that is associated with carbohydrate and lipid abnormalities comes from studies of patients with cerebral vascular disease. Both abnormal glucose tolerance and elevation of serum cholesterol and triglyceride levels were found in the majority of patients and in only a few control subjects[55,56].

EPIDEMIOLOGICAL STUDIES

Although there is persuasive evidence from clinical and autopsy studies that there is an association between atherosclerosis and diabetes, the strongest evidence of the association comes from studies in populations. Population studies have addressed two questions. One is the association between diabetes and atherosclerosis and its consequences, and the other the question of whether blood sugar abnormalities too minor to be designated diabetic are also associated with atherosclerosis. In addition, other factors including age and sex, and risk factors such as hypertension, have been studied and their interaction with both diabetes and atherosclerosis investigated.

Two important studies of diabetes and atherosclerosis were carried out in Bedford, England[57] and Tecumseh, Michigan[58,59]. In the Bedford study known diabetics were excluded. The blood sugar was measured 2 h after 50 g glucose in a group of subjects who had glycosuria and a matched group of controls. On the basis of the blood sugar results the subjects were classified as diabetic, where the blood sugar was more than 200 mg/dl, borderline where the blood sugar was 120–199 mg/dl, and normal where the blood sugar was 119 mg/dl or less. The prevalence of atherosclerosis was assessed by examination of the ECG and by a questionnaire on symptoms. It was found that in both males and females there was a progressive increase in the prevalence of arterial disease with increasing blood sugar (Table 3.6).

Table 3.6 Prevalence of arterial disease (percentages) in relation to blood sugar – Bedford, England[57]

Age (years)	Blood sugar 2 h after 50 g glucose		
	< 120 mg/dl	120–199 mg/dl	> 200 mg/dl
< 50	17	29	41
50–59	24	40	37
60–69	49	68	39
70 and over	45	56	76

This occurred in all ages and was not influenced by blood pressure. Later studies in the same population showed that the incidence of cardiovascular disease over a 5-year period was similarly related to the blood sugar levels[60]. In Tecumseh[58,59] 60% of the subjects had glucose tolerance tests while others had a casual blood sugar measured. Those whose sugars were above the 80th centile were designated hyperglycaemic and to these were added the known diabetics. At all ages, the number of cardiovascular events was greater in the diabetics than in the population as a whole (Table 3.7). Similarly hyperglycaemia was found in a higher proportion of subjects with atherosclerotic disease than in the population as a whole. It was

Table 3.7 (a) Prevalence of vascular disease in diabetics – Tecumseh, Michigan (observed: expected)[59]

Age (years)	Male	Female
40–59	3.3	2.7
60+	1.6	1.7
TOTAL	1.9	1.8

(b) Prevalence of hyperglycaemia (blood sugar more than 80th centile plus known diabetics) among persons with vascular disease – Tecumseh, Michigan (observed : expected)[59]

Vascular disease	Male	Female
Coronary heart disease	1.7	1.8
Peripheral and cerebral vascular disease	1.5	1.9
T-wave changes	1.8	1.9
Hypertension	1.2	1.4

concluded that hyperglycaemia had an independent relationship with coronary heart disease even when other risk factors were taken into account[58]. At the 7-year follow-up of the Tecumseh population[61] the incidence of myocardial infarction or death was increased in all subjects with glucose intolerance except men aged 50–64. The relationship was independent of blood pressure. At the 1977 examination[62] subjects who developed coronary heart disease had a significantly higher mean blood glucose concentration than other members of the cohort even after exclusion of known diabetics. Other variables including age, sex, systolic blood pressure, relative body weight, serum cholesterol and the number of cigarettes smoked per day were also more frequent in the subjects who had developed coronary heart disease. However, when multiple logistic analysis was carried out only age, degree of smoking, blood pressure and blood glucose were significant variables. Glucose and cholesterol significantly interacted but the interaction lost its significance when known diabetics were excluded. The risk ratio for coronary heart disease was calculated from the number of observed coronary events in the upper quartile of distribution of projected risk divided by the observed number of events in the lowest quartile. In the whole group the risk ratio for blood glucose was 2.2, and when the eleven subjects with diabetes were excluded, this fell to 2.1. The Tecumseh studies thus indicate that hyperglycaemia and diabetes are associated with an increased prevalence and incidence of coronary artery disease which was still present when subjects with diagnosed diabetes were excluded. The close interaction between blood glucose and other risk factors for atherosclerosis makes the exact relationship between blood glucose and vascular disease complex.

Another important population study was carried out in an industrial community[63]. In the initial prevalence study of 1356 subjects it was found that those diagnosed as diabetic on clinical grounds had a 2.5 times greater rate of myocardial infarction than those who were not diabetic. In a later prevalence study in the same population but involving 1963 subjects, those with diabetes had a higher prevalence of atherosclerotic heart disease, myocardial infarction and hypertension than controls. Peripheral vascular disease, although twice as frequent in the diabetics, was uncommon and the difference was not significant[64]. A high prevalence of hypertension was noted in the diabetics. However, although the prevalence of atherosclerotic heart disease was higher in the hypertensive men whether or not they were diabetic, diabetes increased the prevalence of atherosclerotic disease whether the blood pressure was normal or raised.

The factors associated with mortality and survival of diabetics were assessed in the same population[65]. The 10-year survival of diabetics was 74.6% whereas that for non-diabetics was 90.3%. The death rate in diabetics was greater at all ages although the excess risk fell with increasing age. Hypertension conferred no greater risk in diabetics than in controls and the mortality rate rose with increasing weight in both diabetics and controls. Atherosclerotic heart disease was a much commoner cause of death in diabetics than in non-diabetics. The mortality from coronary heart disease was also higher in the diabetics (13.2%) than in the non-diabetics (4.6%). The mortality from coronary heart disease increased with both the dose of insulin and the amount of glycosuria, suggesting that it was influenced by the severity of diabetes (Table 3.8). Overall, this study suggests that the risk factors for atherosclerosis operate in diabetics as in non-diabetics and do not entirely account for the increased risk of atherosclerosis in the diabetics.

Table 3.8 Mortality in diagnosed diabetics in relation to age, daily dose of insulin and glycosuria (ratio of deaths in diabetics to deaths in non-diabetics)[65]

	Age (years)			Dose of insulin (units)			Glycosuria		
	<45	45–54	55–64	0	<40	40+	0–1	2–3	4–5
Mortality rate	6.7	2.7	2.0	2.2	2.5	5.7	2.1	2.7	4.1

The major epidemiological study of risk factors in atherosclerosis has been the Framingham study. In this large prospective study of 5209 men and women, diabetes was diagnosed on clinical grounds when the patient was having treatment for diabetes, had an impaired oral glucose tolerance test or had two or more blood glucose levels higher than 160 mg/dl. The relationship of blood glucose to vascular disease was first reported at the 16th year of the study[66]. At that time diabetic men and women had developed more cerebrovascular accidents, coronary heart disease and peripheral arterial disease than age- and sex-matched non-diabetics. The mortality rate in diabetic women was $4\frac{1}{2}$ times that in non-diabetic women but in men the risk ratio was about 2:1. Diabetes removed the protective effect of the female sex in the development of atherosclerosis. However, the excess frequency of vascular disease in women was confined to those who were treated with insulin. Coronary disease was the commonest cause of death in the diabetics but the impact of diabetes appeared to be greatest on intermittent claudication. Although the diabetics had higher serum cholesterol levels, blood pressure and relative weight than the non-diabetics the differences were not considered to be of sufficient magnitude to account entirely for the excess of atherosclerotic vascular disease in the diabetics. Multivariate analysis of the risk factors showed that there appeared to be some unique effect of diabetes, especially in women, which could not be explained by associated risk factors. The results of later examinations of the Framingham population have confirmed the findings of the 16-year examination[67]. In particular the increased risk of cardiovascular disease in young women was confirmed (Table 3.9). Diabetes is not a highly

Table 3.9 Risk ratios for cardiovascular disease in diabetics in relation to age and sex

Age (years)	Men	Women
45–54	2.7	6.3
55–64	1.9	2.9
65–74	2.1	1.8
All ages	2.1	2.7

The risk ratio is the ratio of the incidence in diabetics to that in non-diabetics (the Framingham Study[68])

prevalent condition and when considered in relation to the other risk factors for atherosclerosis, diabetes carries a relatively low risk[68]. Other risk factors such as hypertension and serum cholesterol were found to have the same relationship to cardiovascular disease in diabetics as in non-diabetics and there was no evidence that diabetics cope less well with risk factors than non-diabetics[69]. HDL are thought to have a protective effect on the development of atherosclerosis but even when the HDL values were taken into consideration the impact of diabetes on cardiovascular disease could not be entirely explained by the associated risk factors[70].

BLOOD SUGAR AND ATHEROSCLEROSIS

Some recent studies have addressed the question as to whether blood sugar elevations in the absence of manifest diabetes are related to atherosclerosis. A group of investigators from a number of different countries published their results together as the International Collaborative Project[71]. This was not a collaborative study designed in advance and there were differences in the design and execution of the different studies. An increased risk of cardiovascular disease in subjects with the highest blood glucose levels was found in only four of the studies. It was concluded that overall there was insufficient evidence to suggest that hyperglycaemia was a significant independent risk factor for atherosclerosis or that it had a threshold effect; in other words, that there was a blood glucose level above which atherosclerosis became more common. It was suggested that hyperglycaemia should not be designated an independent risk factor for coronary heart disease (CHD) on present evidence.

There are a number of problems with the International Collaborative Project[72]. One is that the studies included in the project differed in a number of respects including methods of measuring blood glucose, times at which samples were taken for the measurement of glucose, and certain exclusion criteria for patients with pre-existing diabetes. Differences between populations are also possible. The studies which showed an excessive CHD mortality with the highest blood sugar levels were the only studies in which a significant number of coronary deaths occurred in subjects with the highest blood sugar levels. Indeed, only four of the studies had more than one CHD death in the upper blood sugar quintile and of these three showed at least a doubling of mortality in this blood sugar range. One of the studies included in this project was the Whitehall study, a prospective study of 18 403 civil servants and by far the largest study in the group. Later results from this study have been published separately[73]. Capillary blood sugar was measured 2 h after a 50 g oral glucose load had been administered after an overnight fast. Subjects were classified as diabetic, i.e. those who were previously diagnosed as diabetic; new diabetics, i.e. those whose 2 h blood sugar level was 200 mg/dl or more; and the remainder. The diabetic subjects had high mortality rates and the highest prevalence of ECG abnormalities. The highest mortality rate was found in subjects with 2 h blood sugar levels more than 200 mg/dl, in other words, those designated as new diabetics. In those whose 2 h blood sugar level was less than 200 mg/dl a linear relationship between blood glucose and the age-adjusted CHD mortality or the prevalence of ECG abnormalities was not found. However, there was a sharp doubling of the 7½-year CHD mortality at the 95th centile (2 h blood sugar 96 mg/dl).

It is notable that in the Whitehall study the increased risk of CHD mortality and ECG abnormalities was found at blood sugar levels which are considerably lower than those recently recommended for the diagnosis of impaired glucose tolerance[6]. The findings also contrast with those reported for microvascular disease in diabetes as manifest by retinopathy and proteinuria. In the Pima Indians of Arizona, a community with the highest recorded prevalence of diabetes, the development of retinopathy in a 3-year period was very rare in those with a fasting blood sugar of less than 140 mg/dl and did not occur if the 2 h blood glucose was less than 200 mg/dl[74]. Proteinuria was less frequent than retinopathy but had a similar relationship to blood glucose levels.

The Whitehall findings are consistent with those of the Tecumseh study which also found a doubling of CHD incidence in those with the highest blood sugar levels when diabetics were excluded. The exact nature of this threshold relationship of blood glucose to atherosclerosis is unclear. Nevertheless, if the relationship is confirmed it can explain why linear relationships between blood glucose and atherosclerosis have not been found in certain other studies. It is possible that blood glucose levels above a critical point have metabolic actions which predispose to atherosclerosis. These actions may be on the arterial wall itself, or may act via other aspects of carbohydrate or lipid metabolism. On the other hand those with the higher blood glucose levels may be genetically predisposed to diabetes and to atherosclerosis and have an underlying cellular defect which predisposes to vascular disease. The relationship of blood glucose and atherosclerosis to other risk factors for atherosclerosis also must be considered.

DIABETES AND SILENT MYOCARDIAL INFARCTION

It is often stated that myocardial infarction and ischaemic heart disease is more frequently associated with the absence of pain in diabetics than in non-diabetics[75]. The Framingham study has addressed this question, and both their 14-year follow-up[76] and their 18-year follow-up[77] found that diabetics were approximately twice as likely as non-diabetics to have silent myocardial infarctions. The number of silent myocardial infarctions was of course small and the relationship with diabetes did not reach statistical significance. In the Israeli ischaemic heart disease study, unrecognized myocardial infarction was related to age but not to diabetes[78]. Further studies of larger numbers of patients with silent myocardial infarction will be needed before this question can be satisfactorily resolved.

CONCLUSIONS

Evidence from autopsy, clinical and epidemiological studies is overwhelmingly in favour of the proposition that atherosclerosis is more advanced in diabetics than non-diabetics. While diabetes may be associated with some other risk factors for atherosclerosis, hyperglycaemia is an independent risk factor for cardiovascular disease. Nevertheless, cardiovascular disease incidence is not linearly related to the blood sugar level, nor is it related to the duration or severity of diabetes or the method of treatment. Recent population studies have suggested that there is a threshold relationship between blood sugar and cardiovascular disease, the incidence of the disease rising rapidly when the blood sugar is higher than a certain level. This may indicate that hyperglycaemia has harmful effects on arteries or that a population with an increased susceptibility to atherosclerosis, perhaps genetically based, has been identified.

References

1. Marks, H. H. and Krall, L. F. (1971). Onset course, prognosis and mortality in diabetes mellitus. In Marble, A., White, P., Bradley, R. F. and Krall, L. F. (eds.) *Joslin's Diabetes Mellitus*, pp. 209-54. (Philadelphia: Lea & Febiger)
2. West, K. M. (1978). *Epidemiology of Diabetes and its Vascular Lesions*. (New York: Elsevier)
3. Stout, R. W., Bierman, E. L. and Brunzell, J. D. (1975). Atherosclerosis and disorders of lipid metabolism in diabetes. In Vallance-Owen, J. (ed.) *Diabetes: its Physiological and Biochemical Basis*, pp. 125-69. (Lancaster: MTP Press)
4. Stout, R. W. (1981). Blood glucose and atherosclerosis. *Arteriosclerosis*, 1, 227
5. Strandness, D. W., Priest, R. W. and Gibbons, G. E. (1964). Combined clinical and pathologic study of diabetic and non-diabetic peripheral arterial disease. *Diabetes*, 13, 336
6. WHO Expert Committee on Diabetes Mellitus (1980). Second Report, World Health Organization Technical Report Series 646
7. Fitz, R. and Murphy, W. P. (1924). The cause of death in diabetes mellitus. *Am. J. Med. Sci.*, 168, 315
8. Warren, S. and Root, H. F. (1925). The pathology of diabetes, with special reference to pancreatic regeneration. *Am. J. Pathol.*, 1, 415
9. Blottner, H. (1930). Coronary disease in diabetes mellitus. *N. Engl. J. Med.*, 203, 709
10. Root, H. F. and Sharkey, T. P. (1930). Arteriosclerosis and hypertension in diabetes. *Ann. Intern. Med.*, 9, 873
11. Nathanson, M. H. (1932). Coronary disease in 100 autopsied diabetics. *Am. J. Med. Sci.*, 183, 495
12. Root, H. F., Bland, E. F., Gordon, W. H. and White, P. D. (1939). Coronary atherosclerosis in diabetes mellitus. *J. Am. Med. Assoc.*, 113, 27
13. Robbins, S. L. and Tucker, A. W. (1944). The cause of death in diabetes. *N. Engl. J. Med.*, 231, 865
14. Stearns, S., Schlesinger, M. J. and Rudy, A. (1947). Incidence and clinical significance of coronary artery disease in diabetes mellitus. *Arch. Intern. Med.*, 80, 463
15. Editorial (1948). Diabetes – a mass experiment in the study of arteriosclerosis. *N. Engl. J. Med.*, 238, 412
16. Clawson, B. J. and Bell, E. T. (1949). Incidence of fatal coronary disease in nondiabetic and diabetic persons. *Arch. Pathol.*, 48, 105
17. Feldman, M. and Feldman, M. Jr. (1954). The association of coronary infarction and occlusion with diabetes mellitus. A necropsy study. *Am. J. Med. Sci.*, 228, 53
18. Liebow, I. M., Hellerstein, H. K. and Miller, M. (1955). Arteriosclerotic heart disease in diabetes mellitus. *Am. J. Med.*, 18, 438
19. Breithaupt, D. J. and Leckie, R. B. (1961). Diabetes mellitus: a study of the practicability of life insurance. *Can. Med. Assoc. J.*, 85, 299
20. Robertson, W. B. and Strong, J. P. (1968). Atherosclerosis in persons with hypertension and diabetes mellitus. *Lab. Invest.*, 18, 538
21. Mitchell, J. R. A. and Schwartz, C. J. (1965). *Arterial Disease*. (Oxford: Blackwell)
22. Waller, B. F., Palumbo, P. J., Lie, J. T. and Roberts, W. C. (1980). Status of the coronary arteries at necropsy in diabetes mellitus with onset after age 30 years. *Am. J. Med.*, 69, 498
23. Vigorita, V. J., Moore, G. W. and Hutchins, G. M. (1980). Absence of correlation between coronary arterial atherosclerosis and severity or duration of diabetes mellitus of adult onset. *Am. J. Cardiol.*, 46, 535
24. Crall, F. V. and Roberts, W. C. (1978). The extramural and intramural coronary arteries in juvenile diabetes mellitus. Analysis of nine necropsy patients aged 19–38 years with onset of diabetes before age 15 years. *Am. J. Med.*, 64, 221
25. Levine, S. A. (1922). Angina pectoris – some clinical considerations. *J. Am. Med. Assoc.*, 79, 928

26. Nathanson, W. M. (1925). Disease of the coronary arteries. *Am. J. Med. Sci.*, **170**, 240
27. Kahn, M. H. (1926). Etiologic factors in angina pectoris. *Am. J. Med. Sci.*, **172**, 195
28. Levine, S. A. (1929). Coronary thrombosis: its various clinical features. *Medicine*, **8**, 245
29. Connor, L. A. and Holt, E. (1930). The subsequent course and prognosis in coronary thrombosis. *Am. Heart J.*, **5**, 705
30. Master, A. M., Dack, S. and Jaffe, H. L. (1939). Age, sex and hypertension in myocardial infarction due to coronary occlusion. *Arch. Intern. Med.*, **64**, 767
31. Aarseth, S. (1953). Cardiovascular renal disease in diabetes mellitus. *Acta Med. Scand.*, suppl. 281
32. Bartels, C. C. and Rullo, F. R. (1958). Unsuspected diabetes mellitus in peripheral vascular disease. *N. Engl. J. Med.*, **259**, 633
33. Sievers, J., Blomqvist, G. and Biorck, G. (1961). Studies on myocardial infarction in Malmo, 1935 to 1954; VI. Some clinical data with particular reference to diabetes, menopause and heart rupture. *Acta Med. Scand.*, **169**, 95
34. Fabrykant, M. and Gelfand, M. L. (1964). Symptom-free diabetes in angina pectoris. *Am. J. Med. Sci.*, **247**, 665
35. Conrad, M. C. (1967). Large and small artery occlusion in diabetics and nondiabetics with severe vascular disease. *Circulation*, **36**, 83
36. Datey, K. K. and Nanda, N. C. (1967). Hyperglycemia after acute myocardial infarction. Its relation to diabetes mellitus. *N. Engl. J. Med.*, **276**, 262
37. Bailey, R. R. and Beavan, D. W. (1968). Diabetes mellitus and myocardial infarction. *Aust. Ann. Med.*, **17**, 312
38. Reid, D. D., Brett, G. Z., Hamilton, P. J. S., Jarrett, R. J., Keen, H. and Rose, G. (1974). Cardiorespiratory disease and diabetes among middle aged male civil servants. *Lancet*, **1**, 469
39. Wessler, S. and Silberg. N. R. (1953). Studies in peripheral arterial occlusive disease. II. Clinical findings in patients with advanced arterial obstruction and gangrene. *Circulation*, **7**, 810
40. Waitzkin, L. (1967). Unknown diabetes mellitus among apparently healthy men with nonspecific T wave abnormalities in a mental hospital. *Diabetes*, **16**, 722
41. Raab, A. P. and Rabinowitz, M. A. (1936). Glycosuria and hyperglycemia in coronary thrombosis. *J. Am. Med. Assoc.*, **106**, 1705
42. Goldberger, E., Alesio, J. and Woll, F. (1945). The significance of hyperglycaemia in myocardial infarction. *NY State J. Med.*, **45**, 391
43. Waddell, W. R. and Field, R. A. (1960). Carbohydrate metabolism in atherosclerosis. *Metabolism*, **9**, 800
44. Sowton, E. (1962). Cardiac infarction and the glucose-tolerance test. *Br. Med. J.*, **1**, 84
45. Reaven, G., Calciano, A., Cody, R., Lucas, C. and Miller, R. (1963). Carbohydrate intolerance and hyperlipaemia in patients with myocardial infarction without known diabetes mellitus. *J. Clin. Endocrinol.*, **23**, 1013
46. Reissell, P. K., Poon-King, T. M. W., Hagopian, L. M. and Hatch, F. T. (1964). Abnormal tolerance to glucose and fat loads in young males with coronary heart disease. *Circulation*, **30** (suppl. 3), 24
47. Cohen, A. M. and Shafrir, E. (1965). Carbohydrate metabolism in myocardial infarction. *Diabetes*, **14**, 84
48. Jakobson, T., Kahanpaa, A. and Maenpaa, V. J. (1968). Prednisone–glucose tolerance and serum lipids in survivors of myocardial infarction. *Acta Med. Scand.*, **184**, 451
49. Wahlberg, F. (1966). Intravenous glucose tolerance in myocardial infarction, angina pectoris and intermittent claudication. *Acta Med. Scand.*, **180** (suppl.), 453
50. Wahlberg, F. and Thomasson, B. (1968). Glucose tolerance in ischaemic cardiovascular disease. In Dickens, F., Randle, P. J. and Whelan, W. J. (eds.) *Carbohydrate Metabolism and its Disorders*, pp. 185–98. (London: Academic Press)
51. Heinle, R. A., Fredrickson, D. S., Levy, R. I., Herman, M. V. and Gorlin, R. (1967). Incidence of metabolic abnormalities in angiographically demonstrated coronary artery disease. *J. Clin. Invest.*, **46**, 1069
52. Herman, M. V. and Gorlin, R. (1967). Coronary artery disease and diabetes mellitus. In Hamwi, G. J. and Danowski, T. S. (eds.) *Diabetes Mellitus: Diagnosis and Treatment*, pp. 329–42. (New York: American Diabetes Association)

53. Falsetti, H. L., Schnatz, J. D., Greene, D. G. and Bunnell, I. L. (1968). Lipid and carbohydrate studies in coronary artery disease. *Circulation*, **37**, 184
54. Falsetti, H. L., Schnatz, D. J., Greene, D. G. and Bunnell, I. L. (1968). Carbohydrate and lipid studies in 27 patients with coronary artery disease. *Diabetes*, **16**, 505
55. Jakobson, T. (1967). Glucose tolerance and serum lipid levels in patients with cerebrovascular disease. *Acta Med. Scand.*, **182**, 233
56. Albanese, A. A., Lorenze, E. J. and Orto, L. A. (1968). Effect of strokes on carbohydrate tolerance. *Geriatrics*, **23**, 142
57. Keen, H., Rose, G., Pyke, D. A., Boyns, D., Chlouverakis, C. and Mistry, S. (1965). Blood sugar and arterial disease. *Lancet*, **2**, 505
58. Epstein, F. H., Ostrander, L. D., Johnson, B. J. *et al.* (1965). Epidemiological studies of cardiovascular disease in a total community – Tecumseh, Michigan. *Ann. Intern. Med.*, **62**, 1170
59. Ostrander, L. D., Francis, T., Hayner, N. S., Kjelsberg, M. O. and Epstein, F. H. (1965). The relationship of cardiovascular disease to hyperglycemia. *Ann. Intern. Med.*, **62**, 1188
60. Jarrett, R. J. (1971). Diabetes, hyperglycaemia and arterial disease. *Acta Diabet. Lat.*, **8** (suppl. 1), 7–11
61. Epstein, F. H. (1973). Glucose intolerance and cardiovascular disease. *Triangle*, **12**, 3
62. Ostrander, L. D., Lamphiear, D. E., Carman, W. J. and Williams, G. W. (1981). Blood glucose and risk of coronary disease. *Arteriosclerosis*, **1**, 33
63. Pell, S. and D'Alonzo, C. A. (1963). Acute myocardial infarction in a large industrial population. *J. Am. Med. Assoc.*, **185**, 831
64. Pell, S. and D'Alonzo, C. A. (1968). Diabetes in industry. *Arch. Environ. Health*, **17**, 425
65. Pell, S. and D'Alonzo, C. A. (1970). Factors associated with long-term survival of diabetes. *J. Am. Med. Assoc.*, **214**, 1833
66. Garcia, M. J., McNamara, P. M., Gordon, T. and Kannell, W. B. (1974). Morbidity and mortality in diabetics in the Framingham population. Sixteen year follow-up study. *Diabetes*, **23**, 105
67. Gordon, T., Castelli, W. P., Hjortland, M. C., Kannel, W. B. and Dawber, T. R. (1977). Diabetes, blood lipids and the role of obesity in coronary heart disease risk for women. The Framingham study. *Ann. Intern. Med.*, **87**, 393
68. Kannel, W. B. and McGee, D. L. (1979). Diabetes and cardiovascular disease. The Framingham study. *J. Am. Med. Assoc.*, **241**, 2035
69. Kannel, W. B. and McGee, D. L. (1979). Diabetes and cardiovascular risk factors: the Framingham Study. *Circulation*, **59**, 8
70. Kannel, W. B. and McGee, D. L. (1979). Diabetes and glucose tolerance as risk factors for cardiovascular disease: the Framingham study. *Diabetes Care*, **2**, 120
71. International Collaborative Group (1979). Joint Discussion. *J. Chron. Dis.*, **32**, 829
72. Editorial (1980). Diabetes, hyperglycaemia and coronary heart disease. *Lancet*, **1**, 345
73. Fuller, J. H., Shipley, M. J., Rose, G., Jarrett, R. J. and Keen, H. (1980). Coronary-heart-disease risk and impaired glucose tolerance. *Lancet*, **1**, 1373
74. Pettitt, D. J., Knowler, W. C., Lisse, J. R. and Bennett, P. H. (1980). Development of retinopathy and proteinuria in relation to plasma–glucose concentrations in Pima Indians. *Lancet*, **2**, 1050
75. Bradley, R. F. and Schonfeld, A. (1962). Diminished pain in diabetic patients with acute myocardial infarction. *Geriatrics*, **17**, 322
76. Kannel, W. B., McNamara, P. N., Feinbach, M. and Dawber, T R. (1970). The unrecognised myocardial infarction. Fourteen-year follow-up experience in the Framingham study. *Geriatrics*, **25**, 75
77. Margolis, J. R., Kannel, W. B., Feinleib, M., Dawber, T. R. and McNamara, P. M. (1973). Clinical features of unrecognised myocardial infarction – silent and symptomatic. *Am. J. Cardiol.*, **32**, 1
78. Medalie, J. H. and Goldbourt, U. (1976). Unrecognised myocardial infarction: five year incidence, mortality and risk factors. *Ann. Intern. Med.*, **84**, 526
79. Goodkin, G. (1975). Mortality factors in diabetes. A 20-year mortality study. *J. Occup. Med.*, **17**, 716

4
Risk factors for atherosclerosis in diabetes

Atherosclerosis occurs more often and at an earlier age in diabetics than in non-diabetics. A possible explanation for this is that risk factors for atherosclerosis in the general population are more common in diabetics. This chapter discusses the prevalence of cardiovascular risk factors in diabetes and their relationship to atherosclerosis in diabetics. Some characteristics of diabetes itself will also be discussed. Abnormalities of lipid metabolism in diabetes are the subject of another chapter.

AGE

The most potent risk factor for atherosclerosis in the general population is increasing age. In diabetes the incidence of atherosclerosis also increases with advancing age. There is evidence that atherosclerosis occurs at a younger age in diabetics than in non-diabetics. Thus it appears that the presence of diabetes accelerates the normal relationship of age to atherosclerosis.

FEMALE SEX

In younger age groups in the general population females are relatively protected against atherosclerosis (Chapter 9). However, this is not the case in diabetics in whom both non-fatal and fatal atherosclerosis is relatively more frequent in females than in males[1] (Table 4.1). The result of this is that the incidence of vascular disease in diabetics is the same in males and females at all ages. In Framingham the impact of diabetes on atherosclerosis in females was most marked in those who were treated with insulin[1]. Presumably these were insulin-dependent diabetics with a fairly severe degree of diabetes. Diabetes is the only condition in which the incidence of atherosclerosis is the same in females as in males at all ages. The explanation of the loss of protection against atherosclerosis in female diabetics is unknown.

Table 4.1 Annual incidence of cardiovascular disease in diabetics aged 45–74 years in the Framingham 20-year follow-up[2]

	Men	Women
Cardiovascular disease	2.0	2.7
Cardiovascular death	2.0	4.7
Congestive heart failure	2.2	5.2
Intermittent claudication	3.8	3.6
Stroke	2.5	3.6
Coronary heart disease	1.7	2.6

Figures are expressed as a ratio of the incidence in non-diabetics

HYPERTENSION

Hypertension is a major risk factor for atherosclerosis and for death from cardiovascular disease[3]. The risk progressively increases with increasing blood pressure and has been shown to be diminished by therapeutic reduction of blood pressure[4,5]. The cardiovascular disorders most closely associated with hypertension are cerebral vascular disease and cardiac failure, the relationship between hypertension and coronary atherosclerosis being less marked.

There is disagreement on the relationship of blood pressure to diabetes and to diabetic vascular disease. A number of studies have shown that blood pressure is somewhat higher in diabetics. For example, the Framingham study[1,6] found hypertension to be slightly more common in both men and women with diabetes (Table 4.2). Similar results were found in the Israeli heart study[7] and the Tecumseh study[8]. In a large industrial study[9] there was a 54% excess of hypertension in diabetics of all ages and both sexes. Review of the records showed that hypertension was often present before the onset of the diabetes and was not related to overweight or to clinical evidence of renal disease. On the other hand, a careful study of diabetics in which the blood pressure was taken at rest and under standardized conditions found no systematic or marked difference in blood pressure between diabetics and matched controls[10]. Diabetics who had evidence of renal disease tended to have higher blood pressure although whether this was cause or effect was not clear. On the other hand, diabetic autonomic neuropathy tended to lower the blood pressure, balancing the effects of renal disease.

The relationship of elevated blood pressure to atherosclerosis in diabetes is also controversial. Multivariate analysis in the Framingham study indicated that although raised blood pressure increased the risk of atherosclerosis in both diabetics and non-diabetics, the increased frequency of atherosclerosis in diabetics could not be accounted for by the rise in

Table 4.2 Cardiovascular risk factors in diabetics and total population (percentage abnormal) in the Framingham Study[1]

	Men		Women	
	Diabetics	Whole population	Diabetics	Whole population
Serum cholesterol (≥ 250 mg/dl)	28.6	27.0	48.0	38.1
Hypertensive (≥ 160/95)	28.0	21.1	24.0	22.3
Relative weight (≥ 120%)	20.5	9.8	42.1	18.9

blood pressure, nor was there any evidence that blood pressure had a more deleterious effect in diabetics than in non-diabetics[11]. Similarly, although the industry study first suggested that the risk of atherosclerotic heart disease was greater in hypertensive diabetics than in normotensive diabetics[9] it was later reported that hypertension had no greater effect on long-term survival in diabetics[12]. The latest analysis from the Tecumseh study[13] showed no significant relationship between systolic blood pressure and blood glucose.

On the other hand, an insurance study[14] suggested that hypertension had a marked effect on mortality in diabetics and that hypertension had a slightly greater effect in diabetics than in non-diabetics, especially in those who were under the age of 40 years. The majority of deaths in the diabetics were related to atherosclerosis. Similarly, a control trial of treatment of border-line diabetes, defined as a blood glucose between 110 mg/dl and 199 mg/dl, 2 h after 50 g of oral glucose, showed that there was a significant relationship between the baseline blood pressure level and the subsequent development of coronary heart disease[15]. In the Whitehall study[16] the risk of coronary death was somewhat higher in hypertensives with impaired glucose tolerance than in those who were normoglycaemic (Table 4.3).

It is difficult to draw conclusions from the differing results of these studies. However, it does seem clear that hypertension is slightly more common in diabetics and that diabetics have slightly higher blood pressure levels than non-diabetics. This may be related to renal disease in diabetics. There is no concurrence that hypertension confers a relatively greater risk of vascular disease in diabetics than in non-diabetics and it is clear that an increased prevalence of hypertension is not the explanation for the high frequency of atherosclerosis in diabetes. Hypertension appears to have a similar influence on the development of atherosclerosis in diabetics as in non-diabetics and its effect appears to be additive to the risk of diabetes.

Table 4.3 7½-year mortality rates by degree of glucose intolerance and risk factor status: the Whitehall Study[16]

	Normo-glycaemic	Impaired glucose tolerance
Cholesterol ⩾ 235 mg/dl	1.8	1.2
Systolic BP ⩾ 153 mmHg	1.8	2.1
Body mass index > 27	1.1	1.4
Current smoker	2.2	1.5
Upper work grade	1.7	1.4
Abnormal ECG	3.8	3.4

Relative risk – presence = absence of risk factors

CIGARETTE SMOKING

Cigarette smoking has been identified as a major risk factor for atherosclerosis in the general population[17]. There is little data on the relationship of cigarette smoking to atherosclerosis in diabetes. There is no evidence that diabetics smoke more than non-diabetics and indeed it has been suggested that they may smoke less[11,18,19]. In the Framingham study[11] the relationship of cigarette smoking to the development of cardiovascular disease was the same in diabetics and non-diabetics. In Tecumseh[13] those who developed coronary heart disease (CHD) smoked almost twice as many cigarettes per day as those who did not. However, there was no interaction between cigarettes smoked and blood glucose, nor did the inclusion of diabetics in the study group influence the relationship of cigarette smoking to CHD. In the Whitehall study[15] there was no relationship between cigarette smoking and the development of CHD in a group of borderline diabetics. Indeed smoking was a slightly less important risk factor for CHD mortality in those who had impaired glucose tolerance than in those who were normoglycaemic[16] (Table 4.3). There is thus no evidence that cigarette smoking explains the excessive development of cardiovascular disease in the diabetics.

OBESITY

The role of obesity in atherosclerosis is controversial. Obesity is associated with a wide variety of metabolic abnormalities including abnormal glucose, insulin and lipid levels. Blood pressure also tends to be higher in those who are obese. Thus any relationship between obesity and atherosclerosis may not be directly related to the excess body weight but to its metabolic accompaniments. This may explain the lack of an independent relationship between obesity and atherosclerosis which has been reported in some studies.

Obesity is considerably more common in diabetics than in the population as a whole[6,11,20] (Table 4.2). Vascular disease is more common in diabetics who have gained weight than in those who have not[21] and diabetics who gained weight but lost it again had a lesser frequency of vascular disease than those who remained overweight. Obesity is more common in diabetics with arterial disease than with those without large vessel complications[22]. The Tecumseh study[13] found a higher relative weight in subjects who developed CHD than those who did not, but also found that relative body weight was not significantly related to CHD in a logistic function analysis. No interaction between body weight and blood glucose was found. Although in the Framingham study[1] weight was higher in diabetic women with cardiovascular disease than in those without, the relationship of body weight to cardiovascular disease did not differ in diabetics and non-diabetics. In the Whitehall study[16] there was no relationship between baseline body mass index and CHD mortality in borderline diabetics but a high body mass index had a stronger relationship to the $7\frac{1}{2}$-year CHD mortality in those with impaired glucose tolerance than in those who were normoglycaemic[16] (Table 4.3).

Obesity is associated with a number of risk factors for atherosclerosis apart from diabetes. Body weight is closely related to circulating triglyceride levels both in diabetics[22] and non-diabetics[23], but triglyceride and obesity seem to be independently related to atherosclerosis in diabetics[22]. The relationship between obesity and triglyceride levels may be mediated by way of the elevated insulin levels associated with obesity[23]. There is also a relationship between body weight and cholesterol levels[24] and obesity is associated with increased total body cholesterol synthesis[25,26]. Hypertension is related to body weight[27,28] and blood pressure is reduced by weight reduction.

The role of obesity in both atherosclerosis itself and in the vascular complications of diabetes is not clear, and any relationship may be indirect. There is little evidence to suggest that obesity may be of greater significance in vascular disease in diabetics than in non-diabetics but further studies specifically directed to this question are required before a definitive answer can be found. It is also not known whether weight reduction will reduce the incidence of vascular disease in either diabetics or non-diabetics. Nevertheless, there are good general reasons for advising against obesity and recommending weight reduction in diabetics who are overweight.

DIET

The relationship of diet to diabetes is complex. There is no evidence that diet plays any role in the development of diabetes except indirectly through its effect on obesity[29,30]. The relationship of diet to the development of CHD is also controversial[31]. Diet influences circulating lipid levels and these may be related to the development of atherosclerosis. The role of diet in the management of diabetes has been subject to recent reappraisal.

There is little published evidence on the relationship of diet to vascular disease in diabetics, and no recent information on this topic. In a retrospective study of diabetics managed two decades apart an increase in the frequency of atherosclerotic complications in the later period was associated with an increase in the carbohydrate content of the diet[32]. Serum triglyceride levels were also higher in the later period and it was suggested that atherosclerosis was related to carbohydrate-induced increases in triglyceride levels. However, more recent studies have failed to find a relationship between dietary carbohydrate and triglyceride levels in diabetics[22] despite a close association between hypertriglyceridaemia and atherosclerosis in these subjects. Furthermore, although increasing the proportion of carbohydrate in the diet induces an acute elevation of circulating fasting triglyceride levels[33], this phenomenon is transient in both diabetics[34,35] and non-diabetics[36] and restricted to the basal (overnight fasted) state. More prolonged studies also showed beneficial effects of high-carbohydrate diets on serum lipids in diabetics with no increase in blood glucose levels[37,38]. Increasing dietary carbohydrate tends to improve glucose tolerance in mild diabetics[39] and lowers fasting glucose levels with no increase in glycosuria or in insulin requirements of insulin-treated diabetics[35,40].

None of the more recent epidemiological and pathological studies of atherosclerosis and diabetes have addressed the question of the relationship of diet to the development of vascular disease. However, in Japan the average diet contains a higher proportion of carbohydrate than in Western countries and the Japanese, whether diabetic or not, tend to have much less atherosclerosis[41]. There have been no reports of prospective studies of diet in the development of vascular disease in diabetes. Thus, the role of diet in pathogenesis of atherosclerosis in diabetics remains unclear.

PHYSICAL ACTIVITY

Physical activity has important effects on carbohydrate metabolism, tending to lower blood glucose levels, increase the efficiency of glucose utilization and hence lower serum insulin levels[42]. The mechanism of this effect has not been clearly worked out and studies of the effect of physical exercise on cell membrane insulin receptors are difficult to interpret because of the concomitant changes in insulin levels. Epidemiological evidence has been presented that vigorous exercise in leisure time protects against CHD[43]. There is very little evidence on the relationship of physical exercise to atherosclerosis in diabetics. A population study in Malmo, Sweden showed that the number of men with impaired glucose tolerance was significantly higher among those who were physically inactive during their leisure time[44]. The Whitehall study[16] made brief reference to physical activity by looking at the work grade of the study subjects. The influence of work grade on the $7\frac{1}{2}$-year mortality was less in those with impaired glucose tolerance than those who were normoglycaemic (Table 4.3).

PLATELETS

The role of thrombosis and coagulation abnormalities in atherosclerosis has been a subject of interest for over a century. The role of platelets and thrombosis in diabetes and atherosclerosis has been recently reviewed[45,46]. Two functions of platelets are used in the development of a platelet clot. The first is adhesion, in which platelets adhere to the arterial wall when the endothelium has been damaged or removed and the subendothelial collagen is exposed. *In vitro* studies using a variety of techniques have indicated that platelet adhesiveness is increased in diabetics of different types with and without vascular disease[46]. The second step is aggregation when the platelets clump together. Platelet aggregation can be measured in the laboratory in the presence of promoting factors. Platelets from diabetics have increased sensitivity to aggregating agents particularly when the diabetics have large- or small-vessel disease[46,47]. Some studies in animals and in humans have indicated that the platelet abnormalities may precede the development of vascular lesions.

Recent research has elucidated some of the biochemical pathways involved in platelet function[48]. The arachidonic acid pathway leads to the production of thromboxane A_2 in the platelet or prostacyclin (PGI) in the endothelial cell. Thromboxane causes platelet aggregation and vasoconstriction while prostacyclin prevents platelet aggregation and causes vasodilation. Abnormalities in these pathways in diabetics would be of considerable interest in relation to atherosclerosis. Increased synthesis of thromboxane B_2, the stable product of the active thromboxane A_2, has been found in platelets from diabetics[49]. Thromboxane synthesis was positively correlated with the plasma glucose at the time of the study. Platelets obtained from diabetic subjects were also less sensitive to anti-aggregatory substances, suggesting the possibility that increased platelet thromboxane synthesis may contribute to enhanced platelet aggregation.

Increased platelet turnover occurs in diabetic subjects with vascular disease and this is accompanied by a high percentage of large platelets (megathrombocytes) in the peripheral blood. These findings suggest that diabetic patients may be depositing platelets *in vivo* leading to increased production of platelets by the bone marrow. Further evidence of increased platelet utilization in diabetics is provided by measurements of plasma beta-thromboglobulin (BTG) a platelet-specific protein. Because BTG has a long half-life it can be used as a guide to platelet utilization *in vivo*. A number of studies have shown elevated plasma levels of BTG in diabetics[46,50,51].

There have been several recent reports of arachidonic acid pathway activity in diabetics (Table 4.4). Three studies measured prostacyclin production by vascular tissue taken from diabetics[52-54] while four reports concern the circulating metabolites of thromboxane A_2 and prostacyclin[55-58]. Vascular tissue prostacyclin production tends to be reduced in diabetics, but there is no agreement on the levels of circulating metabolites. Some studies have attempted to relate the findings to the presence of proliferative retinopathy but none has looked at atherosclerosis. It is not clear whether changes in prostacyclin or thromboxane in diabetic retinopathy are a cause or a result of the microangiopathy. Further studies using larger numbers of well-characterized diabetics are required to investigate the role of the

Table 4.4 Prostacyclin, and prostacyclin and thromboxane A_1 metabolites in diabetics

	No. of diabetics	Type of diabetes	Compli- cations	Vessel	PGI_2
Silberbauer et al. 1979[52]	10	IDDM	?	vein	↓
Johnson et al. 1979[53]	2	IDDM	?	artery	↓
Davis et al. 1981[54]	12	IDDM	6PR	vein	(↓)

	No. of diabetics	Type of diabetes	Compli- cations	6-keto- $PGF_{1\alpha}$	$TBXB_2$
Davis et al. 1979[55]	11	IDDM	no	–	–
Dollery et al. 1979[56]	8	6IDDM	PR	↓	
Davis et al. 1980[57]	28	IDDM	9PR	–	
Yikorkala et al. 1981[58]	53	34IDDM	28PR	↑	↑

IDDM = insulin-dependent diabetes mellitus; PR = proliferative retinopathy; PGI_2 = prostacyclin; 6-keto-$PGF_{1\alpha}$ = 6-keto-prostaglandin $F_{1\alpha}$; $TBXB_2$ = thromboxane B_2; ↓ = decreased in diabetics compared to non-diabetics; ↑ = increased in diabetics; – = no difference between diabetics and non-diabetics; (↓) = non-significant difference.

arachidonic acid pathway in diabetes and atherosclerosis.

Another platelet component is the platelet-derived growth factor, thought to have an important role in the initiation of atherosclerosis[59]. There is no information of the effect of spontaneous or experimental diabetes on the platelet-derived growth factor.

There is evidence suggesting the presence of abnormalities in platelet function in diabetes. Whether these have a role in atherogenesis in diabetes is a topic that requires further study.

GENETIC CONSTITUTION OF DIABETES

In view of the fact that atherosclerosis in diabetes cannot be explained by any of the known risk factors, but that the risk factors appear to be related to atherosclerosis in the same way as in non-diabetics, the possibility that diabetics have a genetic constitution which predisposes to the development of atherosclerosis must be considered. It is possible that groups identified in epidemiological studies such as the Whitehall study, where impaired glucose tolerance is associated with a sharp increase in the frequency of atherosclerosis, may contain those who are genetically predisposed to both diabetes and atherosclerosis.

An attempt to answer this question was made at the 17-year follow-up of the Oxford, Massachussetts study[60]. After diabetics had been excluded it was found that those with the highest postprandial blood glucose levels had the highest chance of developing diabetes. High blood pressure, ECG abnormalities, retinopathy and survival rates were all related to high initial blood glucose levels but not if those who subsequently developed diabetes were excluded. On the other hand, elevated blood glucose levels after oral glucose tolerance tests were also related to hypertension and ECG abnormalities even when subsequent diabetes was excluded. This suggested that those with high blood glucose levels constitute two separate groups. One group is destined to become diabetic but in the other the high blood glucose levels may have a more direct relationship to vascular disease.

Some races and ethnic groups have generally low incidences of cardiovascular disease despite high frequencies of diabetes[61-63]. However, in general the prevalence of cardiovascular disease in diabetics in these populations is higher than that of non-diabetics.

A number of studies have shown abnormalities in skin fibroblasts grown from diabetic donors. Reduced plating efficiency[64], decreased replicative lifespan[65, 66], abnormalities in proliferation and protein synthesis[67], reduced insulin-stimulated leucine incorporation into protein and uridine incorporation into RNA[68], and the synthesis of an abnormal collagen with characteristics of ageing collagen[69] have all been described in diabetic fibroblasts. On the other hand, there were no abnormalities in fibroblasts grown from diabetic Pima Indians with respect to cell density at confluency, plating efficiency, thymidine incorporation, population doubling rates and replicative lifespan[70]. However, the Pima non-diabetics differed from Caucasian non-diabetics in all these features, suggesting that the genetic background of the population is also important. Of particular relevance to atherogenesis, low-density lipoprotein receptor activity was no different in fibroblasts cultured from diabetic donors compared with those from non-diabetics[71] (Figure 4.1).

Results of studies on genetic and cellular abnormalities in diabetes in relation to atherosclerosis are incomplete, and firm conclusions are impossible to make. The available data are consistent with abnormalities in cell function in diabetics. Whether these are related to the pathogenesis of atherosclerosis is not clear. However, if diabetic cells show characteristics of premature ageing[72] this might be related to age-related atherosclerosis. Thus ageing endothelial cells may be less able to repair intimal injury and ageing smooth muscle cells may lose normal growth control[73]. Much further research is required to test these theories. In particular more knowledge of the characteristics of diabetic arterial cells is needed.

SEVERITY, DURATION AND TREATMENT OF DIABETES

The relationship of atherosclerosis to characteristics of the diabetic state itself is difficult to assess. Diabetes is diagnosed on the basis of investigations performed by a doctor, and the diagnosis of diabetes leads

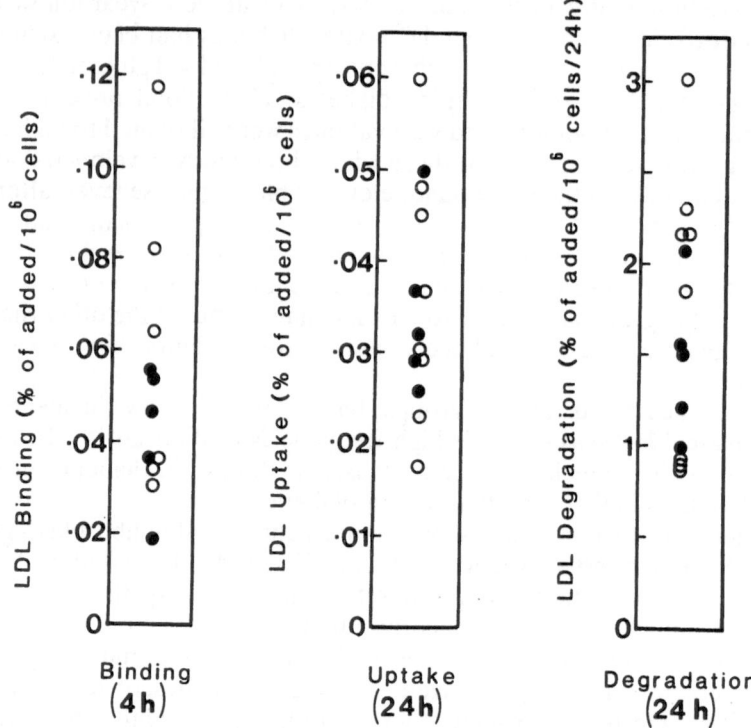

Figure 4.1   Low-density lipoprotein binding uptake and degradation in fibroblasts grown from non-diabetic (●) and diabetic (○) donors[71]

almost invariably to the institution of some form of treatment. The type of treatment prescribed is related to the type of diabetes and to its severity. Thus, it is difficult or impossible in clinical studies to identify the different components of the diabetic state and study them independently.

Studies in the general population including those in Whitehall[16] and Tecumseh[13] show that high blood sugar concentrations in those who are not diabetic or in those who are not previously known to be diabetic are associated with an increased risk of cardiovascular disease, although the risk is not linearly related to the blood sugar level. In those with more severe diabetes the institution of treatment will prevent any study of the relationship of blood sugar levels to development of atherosclerosis.

In most cases it is impossible to determine the date of onset of diabetes. Furthermore, glucose intolerance may be a late manifestation of a complex disorder which may have been present from birth. Atherosclerosis is also a slowly progressive disorder only becoming manifest with advancing years. Thus, both diabetes and atherosclerosis become more common with increasing age and any study of the relationship of the duration of diabetes to atherosclerosis is compounded by the effects of age. A relationship between duration of diabetes and atherosclerosis has been described by some[74-77] but not all authors[78-81]. Other studies have been unable to distinguish the effects of age and duration of diabetes[16,82,83] or found different effects of age and duration in different types of diabetes[84].

The largest study of the relationship of treatment of diabetes to the development of vascular disease is the University Group Diabetes Program Study[85]. This was a randomized controlled trial of five treatment regimes in mild non-insulin-dependent diabetics. The treatments were diet alone, or diet plus tolbutamide, phenformin, a fixed dose of insulin or a dose of insulin which was adjusted to achieve optimal blood glucose lowering. The study reported that no mode of treatment was better than diet alone and suggested that treatment with either tolbutamide[86] or with phenformin[87,88] resulted in an increased mortality from cardiovascular disease. The study has been criticized on a number of grounds[89] and smaller studies with tolbutamine[90,91] and phenformin[15,92] have not confirmed the deleterious effects of these drugs. Nevertheless, it is the only long-term randomized, prospective study of treatment of diabetes and it provides no evidence that treatment reduces the incidence of cardiovascular disease. However, it is also clear from many studies of untreated or newly diagnosed diabetics that vascular disease in diabetes is not solely caused by the treatment used.

Overall there is no convincing evidence that large-vessel disease in diabetes is related to the severity or duration of the disease or is benefited by current therapeutic regimes. This suggests that hyperglycaemia is unlikely to be the main or only causative factor in the development of atherosclerosis in diabetes.

CONCLUSIONS

Atherosclerosis occurs prematurely in diabetics and progresses with advancing age. The normal female protection against atherosclerosis is lost in diabetics of all ages. While hypertension and obesity may be more common in diabetics, they do not explain the increased frequency of atherosclerosis. Cigarette smoking, diet and physical inactivity have no relationship to atherosclerosis in diabetes. While cardiovascular disease is more common in those with high blood sugar levels, the frequency of atherosclerosis in diabetics is unrelated to the severity or duration of diabetes and is not reduced by treatment with insulin or oral hypoglycaemic drugs. Diabetics do not appear to have an increased sensitivity to cardiovascular risk factors.

There is a paucity of information on characteristics which distinguish diabetics with atherosclerosis from those who are free of large-vessel disease. The possibility that combinations of risk factors may be particularly deleterious in diabetics cannot be excluded. However, it appears that there is some unidentified characteristic of the diabetic state that predisposes diabetics to premature atherosclerosis. Whether this is genetic, perhaps some change in cellular growth or metabolism, or secondary to the diabetic state is worthy of further study. The loss of protection against atherosclerosis of female diabetics is another factor whose explanation should be sought.

References

1. Garcia, M. J., McNamara, P. M., Gordon, T. and Kannel, W. B. (1974). Morbidity and mortality in diabetics in the Framingham population. Sixteen year follow-up study. *Diabetes*, **23**, 105
2. Kannel, W. B. and McGee, D. L. (1979). Diabetes and cardiovascular disease. The Framingham study. *J. Am. Med. Assoc.*, **241**, 2035
3. Kannel, W. B. and Dawber, T. R. (1974). Hypertension as an ingredient of a cardiovascular risk profile. *Br. J. Hosp. Med.*, **11**, 508
4. Veterans Administration Co-operative Study Group on Anti-hypertensive Agents (1967). Effects of treatment on morbidity in hypertension. Results in patients with diastolic blood pressure averaging 115 through 129 mm Hg. *J. Am. Med. Assoc.*, **202**, 1028
5. Veterans Administration Co-operative Study Group on Anti-hypertensive Agents (1970). Effects of treatment on morbidity in hypertension. II. Results in patients with diastolic blood pressure averaging 90 through 114 mm Hg. *J. Am. Med. Assoc.*, **213**, 1143
6. Gordon, T., Castelli, W. P., Hjortland, M. C., Kannel, W. B. and Dawber, T. R. (1977). Diabetes, blood lipids, and the role of obesity in coronary heart disease risk for women. The Framingham study. *Ann. Intern. Med.*, **87**, 393
7. Medalie, J. H., Papier, C. M., Goldbourt, U. and Herman, J. B. (1975). Major factors in the development of diabetes mellitus in 10 000 men. *Arch. Intern. Med.*, **135**, 811
8. Ostrander, L. D., Francis, T., Hayner, N. S., Kjelsberg, M. O. and Epstein, F. H. (1965). The relationship of cardiovascular disease to hyperglycemia. *Arch. Intern. Med.*, **62**, 1188
9. Pell, S. and D'Alonzo, C. A. (1967). Some aspects of hypertension in diabetes mellitus. *J. Am. Med. Assoc.*, **202**, 10
10. Keen, H., Track, N. S. and Sowry, G. S. C. (1975). Arterial pressure in clinically apparent diabetics. *Diabete Metab.*, **1**, 159
11. Kannel, W. B. and McGee, D. L. (1979). Diabetes and cardiovascular risk factors: the Framingham study. *Circulation*, **59**, 8
12. Pell, S. and D'Alonzo, C. A. (1970). Factors associated with long-term survival of diabetes. *J. Am. Med. Assoc.*, **214**, 1833
13. Ostrander, L. D., Lamphiear, D. E., Carman, W. J. and Williams, G. W. (1981). Blood glucose and risk of coronary disease. *Arteriosclerosis*, **1**, 33
14. Goodkin, G. (1975). Mortality factors in diabetes. A 20 year mortality study. *J. Occup. Med.*, **17**, 716
15. Jarrett, R. J., Keen, H., Fuller, J. H. and McCartney, M. (1977). Treatment of borderline diabetes: controlled trial using carbohydrate restriction and phenformin. *Br. Med. J.*, **2**, 861
16. Fuller, J. H., Shipley, M. J., Rose, G., Jarrett, R. J. and Keen, H. (1980). Coronary-heart-disease risk and impaired glucose tolerance. *Lancet*, **1**, 1373
17. Gordon, T. and Kannel, W. B. (1972). Predisposition to atherosclerosis in the head, heart, and legs. The Framingham study. *J. Am. Med. Assoc.*, **221**, 661
18. Armstrong, B. and Doll, R. (1975) Bladder cancer mortality in diabetics in relation to saccharin consumption and smoking habits. *Br. J. Prev. Soc. Med.*, **29**, 73
19. Czyzyk, A. and Krolewski, A. S. (1976). Is cigarette smoking more frequent among insulin treated diabetics? *Diabetes*, **25**, 717
20. Pyke, D. A. and Please, N. W. (1957). Obesity, parity and diabetes. *J. Endocrinol.*, **15**, xxvi
21. Reinheimer, W., Bliffen, G., McCoy, J., Wallace, D. and Albrink, M. J. (1967). Weight gain, serum lipids and vascular disease in diabetics. *Am. J. Clin. Nutr.*, **20**, 986
22. Santen, R. J., Willis, P. W. and Fajans, S. S. (1972). Atherosclerosis in diabetes mellitus. *Arch. Intern. Med.*, **130**, 833
23. Bagdade, J. D., Bierman, E. L. and Porte, D. Jr. (1971). Influence of obesity on the relationship between insulin and triglyceride levels in endogenous hypertriglyceridemia. *Diabetes*, **20**, 664
24. Montoye, H. J., Epstein, F. H. and Kjelsberg, M. O. (1966). Relationship between serum cholesterol and body fatness, an epidemiological study. *Am. J. Clin. Nutr.*, **18**, 397
25. Nestel, P. J., Whyte, H. M. and Goodman, D. S. (1969). Distribution and turnover of cholesterol in humans. *J. Clin. Invest.*, **48**, 982

26. Miettinen, T. A. (1971). Cholesterol production in obesity. *Circulation*, **44**, 842
27. Kannel, W. B., Brand, N., Skinner, J. J., Dawber, T. R. and McNamara, P. M. (1967). The relation of adiposity to blood pressure and development of hypertension. The Framingham study. *Ann. Intern. Med.*, **67**, 48
28. Chiang, B. N., Perlman, L. V. and Epstein, F. H. (1969). Overweight and hypertension. *Circulation*, **39**, 403
29. Bierman, E. L. (1979). Carbohydrate and sucrose intake in the causation of atherosclerotic heart disease, diabetes mellitus and dental caries. *Am. J. Clin. Nutr.*, **32**, 2644
30. Medalie, J. H., Papier, C., Herman, J. B. *et al.* (1974). Diabetes mellitus among 10,000 adult men. I. Five year incidence and associated variables. *Israel J. Med. Sci.*, **10**, 681
31. Ahrens, E. H. (1979). Dietary fats and coronary heart disease: unfinished business. *Lancet*, **2**, 1345
32. Albrink, M. J., Lavietes, P. H. and Man, E. B. (1963). Vascular disease and serum lipids in diabetes mellitus. *Ann. Intern. Med.*, **58**, 305
33. Ahrens, E. H., Hirsch, J., Oette, K., Farquhar J. W. and Stein, Y. (1961). Carbohydrate-induced and fat-induced lipemia. *Trans. Assoc. Am. Phys.*, **74**, 134
34. Bierman, E. L. and Hamlin, J. T. (1961). The hyperlipemic effect of a low-fat, high carbohydrate diet in diabetic subjects. *Diabetes*, **10**, 432
35. Stone, D. B. and Connor, W. E. (1963). The prolonged effects of a low cholesterol, high carbohydrate diet upon the serum lipids in diabetic patients. *Diabetes*, **12**, 127
36. Antonis, A. and Bersohn, I. (1961). The influence of diet on serum triglycerides. *Lancet*, **1**, 3
37. Simpson, R. W., Mann, J. I., Eaton, J., Moore, R. A., Carter, R. and Hockaday, T. D. R. (1979). Improved glucose control in maturity-onset diabetes treated with high-carbohydrate-modified fat diet. *Br. Med. J.*, **1**, 1753
38. Simpson, R. W., Mann, J. I., Eaton, J., Carter, R. D. and Hockaday, T. D. R. (1979). High-carbohydrate diets and insulin-dependent diabetics. *Br. Med. J.*, **2**, 523
39. Brunzell, J. D., Lerner, R. L., Hazzard, W. R., Porte, D., Jr and Bierman, E. L. (1971). Improved glucose tolerance with high carbohydrate feeding in mild diabetes. *N. Engl. J. Med.*, **284**, 521
40. Brunzell, J. D., Lerner, R. L., Porte, D., Jr and Bierman, E. L. (1974). Effect of a fat-free, high carbohydrate diet on diabetic subjects with fasting hyperglycemia. *Diabetes*, **23**, 138
41. Keen, H. and Jarrett, R. J. (1973). Macroangiopathy – its prevalence in asymptomatic diabetes. *Adv. Metab. Dis.*, Suppl 2, 3–9
42. Vranic, M. and Berger, M. (1979). Exercise and diabetes mellitus. *Diabetes*, **28**, 147
43. Morris, J. N., Everitt, M. G., Pollard, R. and Chave, S. P. W. (1980). Vigorous exercise in leisure-time: protection against coronary heart disease. *Lancet*, **2**, 1207
44. Lindgarde, F. and Saltin, B. (1981). Daily physical activity, work capacity and glucose tolerance in lean and obese normoglycaemic middle-aged men. *Diabetologia*, **20**, 134
45. Bern, M. M. (1978). Platelet functions in diabetes mellitus. *Diabetes*, **27**, 342
46. Colwell, J. A., Lopes-Virella, M. and Halushka P. V. (1981). Pathogenesis of atherosclerosis in diabetes mellitus. *Diabetes Care*, **4**, 121
47. Halushka, P. V., Lurie, D. and Colwell, J. A. (1977). Increased synthesis of prostaglandin E-like material by platelets from patients with diabetes mellitus. *N. Engl. J. Med.*, **297**, 1306
48. Moncada, S. and Vane, J. R. (1979). Arachidonic acid metabolities and the interactions between platelets and blood-vessel walls. *N. Engl. J. Med.*, **300**, 1142
49. Halushka, P. V., Rogers, R. C., Loadholt, C. B. and Colwell, J. A. (1981). Increased platelet thromboxane synthesis in diabetes mellitus. *J. Lab. Clin. Med.*, **97**, 87
50. Ziboh, V. A., Maruta, H., Lord, J., Cagle, W. D. and Lucky, W. (1979). Increased biosynthesis of thromboxane A$_2$ by diabetic platelets. *Eur. J. Clin. Invest.*, **9**, 223
51. Betteridge, D. J., Zahavi, J., Jones, N. A. G., Shine, B., Kakkar, V. V. and Galton, D. J. (1981). Platelet function in diabetes mellitus in relationship to complications, glycosylated haemoglobin and serum lipoproteins. *Eur. J. Clin. Invest.*, **11**, 273
52. Silberbauer, K., Schernthaner, G., Sinzinger, H., Piza-Katzer, H. and Winter, M. (1979). Decreased vascular prostacyclin in juvenile-onset diabetes. *N. Engl. J. Med.*, **300**, 366

53. Johnson, M., Harrison, H. E., Raftery, A. T. and Elder, J. B. (1979). Vascular prostacyclin may be reduced in diabetes in man. *Lancet,* **1,** 325
54. Davis, T. M. E., Bown, E., Finch, D. R., Mitchell, M. D. and Turner, R. C. (1981). In-vitro venous prostacyclin production, plasma 6-keto-prostaglandin $f_{1\alpha}$ concentrations, and diabetic retinopathy. *Br. Med. J.,* **282,** 1259
55. Davis, T. M. E., Mitchell, M. D. and Turner, R. C. (1979). Prostacyclin and thromboxane metabolites in diabetes. *Lancet,* **2,** 789
56. Dollery, C. T., Friedman, L. A., Hensby, C. N. *et al.* (1979). Circulating prostacyclin may be reduced in diabetes. *Lancet,* **2,** 1365
57. Davis, T. M. E., Mitchell, M. D., Dornan, T. L. and Turner, R. C. (1980). Plasma-6-keto-$PGF_{1\alpha}$ concentrations and diabetic retinopathy. *Lancet,* **1,** 373
58. Yikorkala, O., Kaila, J. and Viinikka, L. (1981). Prostacyclin and thromboxane in diabetes. *Br. Med. J.,* **283,** 1148
59. Ross, R. and Vogel, A. (1978). The platelet-derived growth factor. *Cell,* **14,** 203
60. O'Sullivan, J. B., Cosgrove, J. and McCaughan, D. (1968). Blood sugars, vascular abnormalities and survival. The Oxford study after 17 years. *Postgrad. Med. J.,* **44,** 955
61. Prosnitz, L. R. and Mandell, G. L. (1967). Diabetes mellitus among Navajo and Hopi Indians: the lack of vascular complications. *Am. J. Med. Sci.,* **253,** 700
62. West, K. M. (1974). Diabetes in American Indians and other native populations in the New World. *Diabetes,* **23,** 841
63. Ingelfinger, J. A., Bennett, P. H., Liebow, I. M. and Miller, M. (1976). Coronary heart disease in the Pima Indians. *Diabetes,* **25,** 561
64. Goldstein, S., Littlefield, J. W. and Soeldner, J. S. (1969). Diabetes mellitus and aging: diminished plating efficiency of cultured human fibroblasts. *Proc. Natl. Acad. Sci.,* **64,** 155
65. Vracko, R. and Benditt, E. P. (1975). Restricted replicative life-span of diabetic fibroblasts in vitro: its relation to microangiopathy. *Fed. Proc.,* **34,** 68
66. Goldstein, S., Moerman, S. J., Soeldner, J. S., Gleason, R. E. and Barnett, D. M. (1978). Chronologic and physiologic age affect replicative lifespan of fibroblasts from diabetic, prediabetic and normal donors. *Science,* **199,** 781
67. Rowe, D. W., Scarman, B. J., Fujimoto, W. J. and Williams, R. H. (1977). Abnormalities in proliferation and protein synthesis in skin fibroblast cultures from patients with diabetes mellitus. *Diabetes,* **26,** 284
68. Eckel, R. H. and Fujimoto, W. Y. (1981). Insulin-stimulated glucose uptake, leucine incorporation into protein, and uridine incorporation into RNA in skin fibroblast cultures from patients with diabetes mellitus. *Diabetologia,* **20,** 186
69. Schnider, S. L. and Kohn, R. R. (1981). Effects of age and diabetes mellitus on the solubility and nonenzymatic glycosylation of human skin collagen. *J. Clin. Invest.,* **67,** 1630
70. Howard, B. V., Fields, R. M., Mott, D. M., Savage, P. J., Nagulesparan, M. and Bennett, P. H. (1980). Diabetes and cell growth – lack of differences in growth characteristics of fibroblasts from diabetic and non-diabetic Pima Indians. *Diabetes,* **29,** 119
71. Chait, A., Bierman, E. L. and Albers, J. J. (1979). Low density lipoprotein receptor activity in fibroblasts cultured from diabetic donors. *Diabetes,* **28,** 914
72. Goldstein, S. (1971). Analytical review: the pathogenesis of diabetes mellitus and its relationship to biological aging. *Humangenetik (Berlin),* **12,** 83
73. Stout, R. W. (1981). Atherosclerosis and the metabolism of the arterial wall. In Caird, F. I. and Grimley Evans, J. (eds.) *Advanced Geriatric Medicine,* Vol. 1, pp. 141–51. (London: Pitman)
74. Stearns, S., Schlesinger, M. J. and Rudy, A. (1947). Incidence and clinical significance of coronary artery disease in diabetes mellitus. *Arch. Intern. Med.,* **80,** 463
75. Breithaupt, D. J. and Leckie, R. B. (1961). Diabetes mellitus: a study of the practicability of life insurance. *Can. Med. Assoc. J.,* **85,** 299
76. Ricketts, H. T. (1955). The problem of degenerative vascular disease in diabetes. *Am. J. Med.,* **19,** 933
77. Bradley, R. F. and Bryfogle, J. W. (1956). Survival of diabetic patients after myocardial infarction. *Am. J. Med.,* **20,** 207
78. Liebow, I. M., Hellerstein, H. K. and Miller, M. (1955). Arteriosclerotic heart disease in diabetes mellitus. A clinical study of 383 patients. *Am. J. Med.,* **18,** 438

79. Pyke, D. A. (1968). Coronary disease and diabetes. *Postgrad. Med. J.*, **44** (Suppl.), 966
80. Downie, E. and Martin, F. I. R. (1959). Vascular disease in juvenile diabetic patients of long duration. *Diabetes*, **8**, 383
81. New, M. I., Roberts, T. N., Bierman, E. L. and Reader, G. G. (1963). The significance of blood lipid alterations in diabetes mellitus. *Diabetes*, **12**, 208
82. Krolewski, A. S., Czyzyk, A., Janeczko, D. and Kopczynski, J. (1977). Mortality from cardiovascular disease among diabetics. *Diabetologia*, **13**, 345
83. Kessler, I. I. (1971). Mortality experience of diabetic patients. Twenty-six year follow-up study. *Am. J. Med.*, **51**, 715
84. Beach, K. W., Brunzell, J. D., Conquest, L. L. and Strandness, D. E. (1979). The correlation of arteriosclerosis obliterans with lipoproteins in insulin-dependent and non-insulin-dependent diabetes. *Diabetes*, **28**, 836
85. University Group Diabetes Program (1970). A study of the effects of hypoglycaemic agents on vascular complications in patients with adult-onset diabetes. I. Design, methods and baseline results. *Diabetes*, **19** (suppl. 2), 747
86. University Group Diabetes Program (1970). A study of the effects of hypoglycaemic agents on vascular complications in patients with adult-onset diabetes. II. Mortality results. *Diabetes*, **19** (suppl. 2), 789
87. University Group Diabetes Program (1971). Effects of hypoglycaemic agents on vascular complications in patients with adult-onset diabetes. IV. A preliminary report on phenformin results. *J. Am. Med. Assoc.*, **217**, 777
88. University Group Diabetes Program (1975). A study of the effects of hypoglycemic agents on vascular complications in patients with adult-onset diabetes. V. Evaluation of phenformin therapy. *Diabetes*, **24** (suppl. 1), 65
89. Feisntein, A. R. (1971). Clinical biostatistics. VIII. An analytic appraisal of the University Group Diabetes Program (UGDP) study. *Clin. Pharmacol. Ther.*, **12**, 167
90. Keen, H., Jarrett, R. J., Ward, J. D. and Fuller, J. H. (1973). Borderline diabetics and their response to tolbutamide. *Adv. Metab. Dis.*, suppl. 2, 521
91. Paasikivi, J. (1973). Long-term treatment of patients with abnormal intravenous glucose tolerance after myocardial infarction. *Adv. Metab. Dis.*, suppl. 2, 533
92. Tzagournis, M. and Reynertson, R. (1972). Mortality from coronary heart disease during phenformin therapy. *Ann. Intern. Med.*, **76**, 587

5
Lipid metabolism in diabetes

Diabetes and lipid metabolism has been the subject of a number of recent reviews[1-3]. It has been suggested[4] that abnormalities in lipoprotein metabolism can be understood by examining four sites of regulation of plasma lipoprotein transport:

(1) production of triglyceride-rich lipoproteins,
(2) lipoprotein lipase mediated triglyceride removal,
(3) remnant catabolism,
(4) extra-hepatic cholesterol rich lipoprotein catabolism.

These processes are considered in more detail in Chapter 2.

Diabetes has been shown to affect the first two, and the last, of these processes. Abnormalities of remnant catabolism have not been described in diabetes. As insulin is the most important regulator of lipid metabolism, abnormalities can be conveniently described by considering the effect of insulin on triglyceride and cholesterol metabolism.

INSULIN AND LIPID METABOLISM

Triglyceride metabolism

In non-diabetic subjects with normal or elevated lipids there is a correlation between circulating insulin and triglyceride levels[5]. This may be related to obesity which frequently coexists with hypertriglyceridaemia[6] but the correlation is also present in non-obese hypertriglyceridaemic subjects when it may be related to insulin resistance[7]. In familial hypertriglyceridaemia, the correlation between plasma insulin and triglyceride levels is still present but for identical insulin levels hypertriglyceridaemic subjects have higher triglyceride levels than normal subjects[8]. The relationship between insulin and triglyceride levels is lost in mild diabetes[9] and there is no association between insulin and glucagon secretion and the hypertriglyceridaemia of familial dysbetalipoproteinaemia (type III or broad beta disease)[10].

Insulin acts on several different tissues and organs to exert a major influence on triglyceride production and removal from the circulation.

51

Endogenous triglyceride is synthesized in the liver from fatty acid and glucose substrates. Insulin acts directly on the liver to stimulate triglyceride synthesis[11] and in states of prolonged insulin deficiency, hepatic triglyceride synthesis is depressed[12]. However, when insulin deficiency has been of short duration the liver still seems to be able to respond to an increased supply of substrates by enhancing triglyceride synthesis[13]. The availability of free fatty acid substrate for triglyceride synthesis is also regulated by insulin[14,15]. Circulating free fatty acids result from lipolysis of adipose tissue triglyceride stores. This is mediated by the enzyme hormone sensitive lipase whose activity is inhibited by insulin. Hence in states of insulin excess – for example, after a meal – adipose tissue lipolysis is inhibited, whereas in states of starvation when insulin concentrations are low, adipose tissue lipolysis is active and circulating free fatty acid concentrations increase. Thus, on the production side of triglyceride metabolism, insulin has opposing effects, directly stimulating hepatic triglyceride synthesis while at the same time reducing the supply of free fatty acid substrate.

Triglyceride removal from the circulation is under the influence of the enzyme lipoprotein lipase, an enzyme which is quite distinct from the adipose tissue hormone sensitive lipase. Lipoprotein lipase is synthesized and released from adipose tissue and skeletal muscle. Lipoprotein lipase requires the presence of apoprotein C-II for its activation and may be released into the circulation by the intravenous administration of heparin. The synthesis of lipoprotein lipase is under the influence of insulin and in states of insulin deficiency, lipoprotein lipase concentrations are deficient[16-19]. In extreme insulin deficiency lipoprotein lipase is present in abnormally low concentrations and high concentrations of triglyceride with chylomicronaemia appear in the circulation (diabetic lipemia)[20]. This is reversed by insulin administration. In less severe diabetes, there is a more subtle defect of lipoprotein lipase. After a small amount of heparin is given, lipoprotein lipase in apparently normal amounts is released into the circulation. However if a prolonged heparin infusion is administered, lipoprotein lipase concentrations in the circulation rise but then rapidly fall, in contrast to the normal situation where the concentrations are maintained[21]. This has been termed lipoprotein lipase depletion and is reversible by treatment of diabetes.

Thus a number of different mechanisms may be responsible for hypertriglyceridaemia in diabetes, depending on the type of diabetes[22-25]. In states of insulin deficiency there will be direct depression of hepatic triglyceride synthesis which may be compensated by an increase in the supply of fatty acid substrate from adipose tissue, while at the same time triglyceride removal from the circulation will be impaired. In states of insulin excess, as occurs in the obesity which so often accompanies diabetes, hepatic triglyceride synthesis is enhanced. This interpretation is supported by an experimental study carried out in streptozotocin treated rats[12].

The effects of alterations in insulin secretion on triglyceride metabolism are thus complex and represent a balance between opposing effects on substrate availability, hepatic synthesis and lipoprotein lipase related triglyceride removal.

Cholesterol metabolism

The relationship of insulin to cholesterol metabolism has been less actively studied. Early indications that insulin has a role in cholesterol metabolism were obtained when it was shown that the livers of alloxan diabetic rats had depressed cholesterol synthetic activity[26-28], while intraportal infusion of large concentrations of insulin in alloxan diabetic rats resulted in increased incorporation of acetate into cholesterol[29]. A more direct indication that insulin may promote cholesterol synthesis was obtained in studies of insulin-treated rats[30]. Insulin administration resulted in increased incorporation of labelled acetate into aortic free cholesterol. It was later shown that insulin in physiological concentrations stimulates cholesterol synthesis from acetate in cultured rat aortic smooth muscle cells[31]. No effect of insulin was found when mevalonate was used as substrate, suggesting that insulin acts on 3-hydroxy-3-methylglutaryl coenzyme A reductase (HMG-CoA reductase) the rate-limiting enzyme in the cholesterol biosynthetic pathway. A stimulating effect of insulin on cholesterol synthesis in aortic cells has been reported from another laboratory[32] but the exact identity of these cells was not clear. Insulin also stimulates cholesterol synthesis in hepatic tissue[33], where the effect of insulin is also exerted on HMG-CoA reductase. Hepatic HMG-CoA reductase activity of alloxan diabetic rats is low and insulin injections raise the activity to normal[34,35]. In contrast to the findings in the diabetic rat liver, increased HMG-CoA reductase activity has been found in the intestine of diabetic rats[36]. Thus it appears that insulin deficiency has opposing effects on the two major cholesterol synthesizing organs, suppressing hepatic cholesterol synthesis and enhancing intestinal cholesterol synthesis.

In contrast to the findings in isolated tissues, plasma and hepatic cholesterol levels in alloxan diabetic rats were increased, as was the biliary excretion of cholesterol and bile salts[37]. Intestinal absorption of cholesterol was also increased. These changes were returned to normal by insulin. It was suggested that increased intestinal absorption of cholesterol was a major contributor to the increased cholesterol pool.

It is difficult to relate these findings to human diabetes mellitus. Only three detailed studies of cholesterol metabolism have been performed in human diabetes. Cholesterol metabolism was studied in four untreated diabetic Pima Indians with maturity onset diabetes before and after normalization of blood glucose with insulin[38]. Under metabolic ward conditions, cholesterol balance, bile acid secretion and bile acid pool size as well as lipids and lipoproteins were measured. It was found that the cholesterol balance, the bile acid secretion, the bile acid pool size, fasting plasma cholesterol and plasma triglycerides were all reduced by insulin treatment. The results suggest that both the production of cholesterol and the conversion of cholesterol into bile acids were enhanced in diabetic hyperglycaemia as compared to the insulin-treated state. Insulin treatment also increased the degree to which bile was saturated with cholesterol. Many patients with maturity onset diabetes have already one cause of enhanced cholesterol production, namely obesity[39]. This study, in which weight was held constant, suggested that uncontrolled diabetic hyperglycaemia may be an independent and an additional cause of increased cholesterol production. An association between the concentration of plasma triglycerides and the rate of bile acid secretion was noted in this study and has been reported in a number of other clinical situations. This suggests that production of both VLDL triglyceride and bile acids may be linked to cholesterol synthesis which appears to be increased in early uncontrolled diabetes. The data of the study are consistent with the hypothesis that when maturity onset diabetes is poorly controlled, there is a generalized increase in hepatic lipid production. Insulin appears to reverse this accelerated lipid synthesis.

In another detailed study of cholesterol metabolism in diabetes, five diabetics were studied during a period when their diabetes was under poor control and again following control of diabetes with insulin[40]. Bile acid secretion and sterol balance were measured in a similar fashion to the previous study. Blood glucose fell significantly on treatment and weight increased slightly. Plasma cholesterol changed inconsistently when the subjects were brought under good diabetic control and there was no significant change in the mean plasma cholesterol for all five subjects. Plasma triglycerides showed a downward trend but again the mean change was not significant. Bile acid excretion was decreased after control of the diabetes while neutral sterol excretion was increased. These directly opposite changes in sterol excretory products during insulin treatment resulted in total sterol excretion being unchanged in four subjects and significantly increased in one, a subject who had marked hypertriglyceridaemia with chylomicronaemia. Thus two studies using similar methods produced rather different results.

The methods used in these studies are not very suitable for studying cholesterol metabolism in rapidly changing metabolic states. To overcome these problems a method of measuring cholesterol turnover by kinetic analysis of plasma squalene has been devised. In this method, isotopically labelled mevalonic acid is infused intravenously and the appearance and disappearance of endogenously labelled plasma squalene is measured over a 7 h period. This method was used to study five overweight non-insulin-dependent diabetics in poor diabetic control and after control had been improved by treatment with insulin[41]. Insulin treatment resulted in a fall in blood glucose levels and an increase in cholesterol synthesis. This result is consistent with the effect of insulin on isolated tissues, but differs from both the earlier kinetic studies of cholesterol metabolism in diabetes.

A major mechanism in the regulation of cholesterol transport is the cell membrane LDL receptor. LDL binds to the receptor, is internalized and degraded. Insulin enhances binding and degradation of LDL in cultured human skin fibroblasts while glucose has no effect[42,43] (Figure 5.1). The mechanism of insulin's effect seems to be an increase in the number of LDL receptors rather than a change in binding affinity. LDL receptor activity in fibroblasts from diabetic donors responds to insulin in the same way as that in non-diabetic cells[44]. (Figure 4.1).

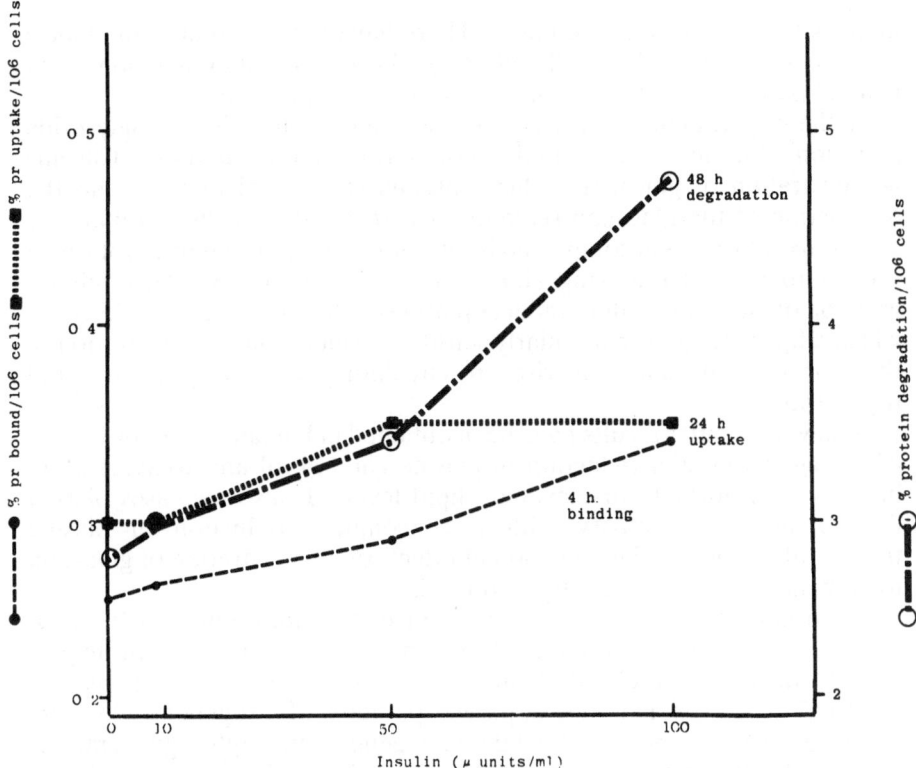

Figure 5.1 Effect of insulin on LDL binding, uptake and degradation in cultured normal human fibroblasts[42]

The evidence available does not allow definite conclusions to be drawn on the effect of diabetes and insulin on cholesterol metabolism. The evidence is consistent with insulin having a stimulating effect on cholesterol synthesis, but also enhancing removal of the main cholesterol carrying lipoprotein by the LDL receptor mechanism. Disorders of insulin secretion will have variable effects on cholesterol transport which is perhaps why plasma cholesterol levels are often normal in diabetes.

The metabolic abnormalities associated with diabetes have complex interrelationships with lipid metabolism and it is difficult to predict the changes that will occur in any particular type of diabetes. Lipoprotein disorders can also occur as a result of genetic abnormalities and a number of different genetic hyperlipidaemias have been described[45]. Diabetes itself has a genetic basis. However, the genetic hyperlipidaemias and diabetes are inherited independently but can occur in the same individual. When this occurs, a severe lipid abnormality is present and lipid levels are not returned to normal by adequate treatment of the diabetes[46].

GLUCAGON AND LIPID METABOLISM

Diabetes is associated with abnormalities in the regulation of glucagon secretion[47]. Glucagon has lipolytic properties in adipose tissue of certain animals but less certainly in man[48]. There have been a number of clinical and experimental studies of the effect of glucagon on lipid metabolism, in general indicating that glucagon reduces plasma lipid levels[49].

In the experimental perfused rat liver, glucagon reduces triglyceride secretion[50] but increases hepatic cholesterol ester formation[51]. Chronic administration of glucagon reduces plasma cholesterol in rats[52] and the destruction of the glucagon secreting pancreatic alpha cells of rabbits by cobaltous chloride is accompanied by elevation of plasma cholesterol which returns to normal following alpha cell regeneration[53]. Similarly administration of glucagon to dogs reduces plasma cholesterol levels[53]. In birds, in which adipose tissue is particularly sensitive to glucagon, administration of the hormone produces a rise in circulating free fatty acids[54] and triglycerides[55].

Somewhat similar results have been obtained in humans. Administration of glucagon causes a reduction in plasma cholesterol and triglyceride in humans with normal[56] or elevated[57] lipid levels. It also increases plasma lipoprotein lipase activity with a concomitant reduction in plasma triglyceride[58]. One of the most potent effects of administration of glucagon to humans is a rise in free fatty acid levels[59].

There have only been a few studies of endogenous glucagon levels in relation to human lipid metabolism. In general subjects with hyper-triglyceridaemia have elevated glucagon levels and glucagon responses to arginine[60,61]. To explain the apparent paradox of exogenous glucagon reducing plasma lipids and while endogenous hyperglucagonaemia is associated with raised plasma triglycerides, it has been suggested that glucagon resistance may occur in human endogenous hyperlipidaemia[62].

The relationship of glucagon to lipid metabolism in diabetes has been little studied. In a study in which physiological elevations of glucagon were attained by glucagon infusion, it was found that in normal subjects the glucagon infusion was accompanied by an increase in endogenous insulin secretion and free fatty acid levels but no effect on plasma triglyceride concentration, while in the diabetics no change in insulin or free fatty acid concentration occurred during the glucagon infusion and circulating triglyceride declined after 20 min of infusion[63].

There is thus evidence that glucagon may have a role in the control of lipid metabolism, and a suggestion that its effects on lipid metabolism may be different in non-diabetic and diabetic subjects. Exogenous glucagon administration results in changes in other hormones and substrates and it is difficult to isolate the contribution of any of these to changes in lipid metabolism. It is likely that changes in glucagon secretion contribute to the lipid abnormalities in diabetes but the exact role of glucagon remains to be elucidated.

LIPID DISORDERS IN DIABETES

The frequency of hyperlipidaemia in diabetes varies in different series. The figures range from 24%[64], 56%[65] and 77%[66] in diabetic children, and 38%[67], 68%[68], 36%[69] and 27%[70] in recent series of diabetic adults. The reasons for the wide variation in the figures are probably selection criteria, definition of hyperlipidaemia, and control and treatment of the diabetes. A recent development in lipoprotein research has been the rediscovery of HDL. The relationship of HDL to diabetes will be considered in detail.

High-density lipoproteins and diabetes

High-density lipoproteins (HDL) have long been ignored in lipoprotein research. This is because of the attention given to the positive association between LDL and atherosclerosis, and because little was known of the origin, function or fate of HDL. Interest in HDL was reawakened in 1975[71] and since then a large amount of investigative work has been carried out on HDL. Epidemiological studies have established a strong negative correlation between plasma HDL cholesterol levels and the risk of developing CHD[72]. The negative correlation between HDL cholesterol and the frequency of CHD occurs in both men and women at all ages studied, and at any level of LDL cholesterol. Decreased HDL levels have also been found in stroke[73,74]. The power of HDL as a negative predictor for atherosclerosis is even greater than the power of LDL as a positive predictor.

There have been a number of studies of HDL in patients with diabetes. The results of these are conflicting and it is difficult to make a definitive statement on HDL in diabetes. The reasons for the differences are not clear although variations in the selection of patients and in laboratory techniques have occurred.

HDL is low in non-insulin-dependent diabetics[75-77] and negatively correlated with blood glucose or HbA_1 in some[75,78] but not all[77] studies. Treatment of diabetes with diet or sulphonylureas restored HDL levels towards normal[75,78]. Differences in HDL in male and female diabetics have also been reported[77]. Pima Indians with non-insulin-dependent diabetes have reduced HDL cholesterol and a low HDL : LDL cholesterol ratio[79].

Insulin-dependent diabetics have raised HDL cholesterol levels[80,81]. HDL was not influenced by diabetic control or body weight[80] and did not correlate with HbA_1 in IDDM[81]. Lipoprotein lipase activity was increased in the insulin-dependent diabetics[80] suggesting that the high HDL levels may have originated in VLDL catabolism. The Framingham study showed normal HDL levels in diabetic men and slightly low levels in diabetic women[82].

A recent study[83] addressed the question as to whether HDL in diabetes might be qualitatively different from that in normals and therefore perhaps predisposed to the development of atherosclerosis. The major constituent apoproteins A-I and A-II were measured in diabetics and controls. HDL cholesterol levels were slightly higher in the diabetics than in the controls and the HDL : LDL cholesterol ratio was significantly higher in diabetic men. The apoprotein A-I : A-II ratio was higher in both diabetic men and diabetic women. This was correlated with HDL_2, a subclass of HDL thought to be most closely involved with reducing the risk of atherosclerosis. Thus HDL composition in diabetics differed from that in non-diabetics in a way which would tend to reduce the risk of developing atherosclerosis.

There is thus no consistent pattern in the results of studies of HDL in diabetes. HDL levels in diabetes are related to the type of diabetes, the presence or absence of obesity, the degree of diabetic control and the type of treatment. Overall it appears that HDL is low in untreated IDDM, but higher than normal when the diabetes is well controlled with insulin. In NIDDM, HDL levels tend to be normal or low depending on the body weight and degree of blood glucose control. It is clear that changes in HDL concentration or composition in diabetes do not consistently predispose to atherosclerosis.

THE EFFECT OF TREATMENT OF DIABETES ON PLASMA LIPIDS

Treatment of diabetes consists of one or more of three measures – modification of the diet, insulin or antidiabetic drugs. There are various ways in which treatment of diabetes would be expected to improve plasma lipid levels. Weight reduction reduces basal hyperinsulinism and hence reduces VLDL synthesis and secretion from the liver[84]. Insulin replacement in insulin-deficient diabetics restores lipoprotein lipase activity to normal and hence improves the removal defect for triglyceride which occurs in these subjects[20,21]. Phenformin lowers both plasma triglyceride and plasma cholesterol. The effect on triglyceride is produced by a reduction in hepatic synthesis of triglyceride probably mediated by reduced glucose, free fatty acid and insulin levels[85]. The effect of sulphonylureas on plasma lipids is less certain but by restoring insulin–glucose relationships towards normal they may have beneficial effects.

For many years the mainstay of dietary treatment of diabetes has been the low-carbohydrate diet. When diabetes is associated with obesity the calorie content of the diet is also restricted. If the carbohydrate content of the diet is decreased, the calorie requirements are made up by increasing the content of fat, usually saturated fat and cholesterol. Recently it has become apparent that the low-carbohydrate and necessarily high-fat diet of the diabetic may contribute to some of the lipoprotein abnormalities.

The effect of dietary composition on plasma lipids and diabetic control has been the subject of a number of studies. In insulin-treated diabetics caloric substitution of carbohydrate for fat in the diet resulted in a fall in serum cholesterol[86]. Contrary to expectation the dietary change did not result in a deterioration of diabetic control. Indeed, in some subjects the insulin dose had to be reduced in order to prevent hypoglycaemia. Other studies have shown similar results. In a study of fasting and diurnal blood lipid levels in 150 young diabetics, it was found that an isocaloric diet rich in polyunsaturated fat resulted in a reduction in blood cholesterol and triglyceride levels[87]. The diet-induced fall in blood lipids was in addition to the lipid-lowering effect of insulin therapy in the untreated juvenile diabetics. The blood sugar level was slightly lower in the group which was given the polyunsaturated fat diet. Another study in diabetic children showed that reduction of cholesterol and saturated fat in the diet resulted in a fall in the prevalence of hyperlipidaemia from 24% on the standard diabetic diet to 5% on the low-fat diet[64]. Preliminary results of a prospective comparison of a low-fat, high-carbohydrate and a low-carbohydrate diet in the treatment of diabetes have been reported from Oxford[88]. The study was carried out in newly diagnosed diabetics not requiring immediate insulin therapy. There was no difference in the effect of the two diets on the fall in blood glucose levels nor on plasma triglyceride. However, the plasma cholesterol decreased on the low-fat, high-carbohydrate diet and this decrease was maintained 1 year after the start of treatment. In mild diabetics high-carbohydrate feeding improves glucose tolerance and reduces fasting plasma glucose levels[89]. Similar benefits of a high-carbohydrate, fat-free diet occur in more severe diabetics who are treated with oral agents or insulin[90,91]. It is suggested that a high-carbohydrate diet increases the sensitivity of peripheral tissues to insulin[89]. Thus it appears that the traditional low-carbohydrate, high-fat diet may be responsible for some of the lipid abnormalities in diabetes. Reducing the fat content of the diet, with a corresponding increase in carbohydrate, results in a lowering of plasma lipids with no decrease, or even an improvement, in diabetic control.

In general, control of fasting glucose levels and glucose tolerance by the use of oral antidiabetic agents or insulin results in a decrease in plasma lipids and a return to normal of plasma lipoprotein patterns[92–97] in most, but not all, diabetics (Table 5.1). Although the persistence of abnormal plasma lipid levels after the institution of diabetic treatment may reflect inadequate diabetic control, it is also possible that some of the patients have coexisting familial lipid disorders[46].

Table 5.1 Lipid, lipoprotein and lipoprotein lipase levels in untreated diabetics, the same diabetics after insulin treatment, and non-diabetic controls[25]

	Diabetics untreated	On insulin	Controls
Lipids (mol/1)			
Serum triglyceride	2.29 ± 0.38	1.15 ± 0.08	0.84 ± 0.07
VLDL-TG	1.59 ± 0.33	0.72 ± 0.09	0.40 ± 0.06
LDL-TG	0.44 ± 0.03	0.28 ± 0.02	0.29 ± 0.02
HDL-TG	0.16 ± 0.09	0.15 ± 0.01	0.15 ± 0.01
Serum cholesterol	6.60 ± 0.4	5.06 ± 0.40	5.40 ± 0.20
VLDL-C	1.08 ± 0.27	0.42 ± 0.06	0.32 ± 0.05
LDL-C	4.41 ± 0.30	3.50 ± 0.20	3.71 ± 0.20
HDL-C	1.11 ± 0.07	1.14 ± 0.07	1.37 ± 0.07
Lipoprotein lipase (μmol FFA l^{-1} g^{-1})			
Adipose tissue LPL	1.09 ± 0.17	1.79 ± 0.32	3.21 ± 0.49
Skeletal muscle LPL	0.42 ± 0.09	0.72 ± 0.39	0.92 ± 0.14

TG = Triglyceride; C = cholesterol; FFA = free fatty acid; other abbreviations as in text

THE RELATIONSHIP OF LIPID ABNORMALITIES TO ATHEROSCLEROSIS IN DIABETES

Although the relationships between diabetes and atherosclerotic vascular disease on the one hand, and between hyperlipidaemia and ischaemic vascular disease on the other, are well established, there is little direct evidence on the question of whether lipid abnormalities connect diabetes and atherosclerosis. One of the earliest studies of this problem showed a relationship between elevated serum triglyceride but not serum cholesterol and CHD in diabetes[98]. The elevated triglyceride levels seemed to be related to dietary intake and weight gain[99]. The closer relationship of triglyceride than cholesterol to diabetic vascular disease was confirmed in later studies[100,101]. In one of the few studies in which diabetics with vascular disease were compared to diabetics without vascular disease it was found that diabetics with evidence of atherosclerosis were more obese and had higher triglyceride and cholesterol levels than those without atherosclerosis[102]. Triglyceride levels were more closely related to atherosclerosis than cholesterol while basal insulin levels, triglyceride levels and body weight were highly interrelated. In Tecumseh[103] a group of subjects who had both cardiovascular disease and hyperglycaemia had significantly higher triglyceride levels than subjects with only one or neither of these abnormalities. Serum cholesterol and blood pressure were similar in all groups in the latest analysis of the Tecumseh data[104]. Serum cholesterol and blood glucose were significantly correlated in the whole group but not when those with diagnosed diabetes were removed from the analysis. In the Whitehall Study the $7\frac{1}{2}$-year mortality from cardiovascular disease had a stronger relationship to raised serum cholesterol levels in normoglycaemic individuals than in those with abnormal glucose tolerance[105]. In the Framingham Study – although other risk factors for atherosclerosis, including lipid abnormalities, occurred in increased frequency in diabetics (Table 5.2) – it was concluded that these alone could not account for the association between diabetes and atherosclerosis[82,106]. On the other hand, low HDL and high LDL concentrations had the same relationship to CHD in diabetics as in non-diabetics (Table 5.3) and there was no evidence that diabetics were more sensitive to risk factors, including lipid abnormalities, than non-diabetics[107,108].

Recently the prevalence of vascular disease in diabetics was analysed in relation to serum lipoprotein concentrations[109]. Diabetics with large-vessel disease had higher total and LDL cholesterol levels and lower HDL cholesterol levels. They also had higher total and VLDL triglyceride levels. When the results were analysed in more detail, vascular disease in the insulin-dependent diabetics was related to elevations in LDL and VLDL but was not related to HDL. In insulin-independent diabetics, higher HDL cholesterol concentrations were related to a reduced prevalence of vascular disease, but there were no significant relationships between vascular disease and the other lipid fractions. In males HDL cholesterol was not related to vascular disease but it was negatively related to vascular disease

Table 5.2 Mean level of certain cardiovascular risk factors in diabetics and non-diabetics: Framingham Study[82]

	Diabetes	No diabetes	p
Men			
HDL-C (mg/dl)	43.9 ± 12.80	46.0 ± 0.46	n.s.
LDL-C (mg/dl)	135.2 ± 3.72	142.4 ± 1.28	n.s.
Triglycerides (mg/dl)	137.9 ± 8.00	135.0 ± 3.48	n.s.
Systolic blood pressure (mmHg)	148.4 ± 2.26	139.1 ± 0.71	<0.001
Relative weight (%)	125.7 ± 1.59	121.5 ± 0.56	<0.05
Women			
HDL-C (mg/dl)	53.5 ± 1.44	57.8 ± 0.44	<0.01
LDL-C (mg/dl)	157.4 ± 3.29	154.5 ± 1.11	n.s.
Triglycerides (mg/dl)	141.3 ± 6.73	113.1 ± 1.67	<0.001
Systolic blood pressure (mmHg)	150.1 ± 2.08	138.8 ± 0.62	<0.001
Relative weight (%)	129.0 ± 1.97	120.6 ± 0.56	<0.001

n.s. = not significant

.**Table 5.3** Incidence of coronary heart disease by diabetic status and level of high-density lipoprotein cholesterol (HDL-C): Framingham Study[82]

HDL-C (mg/dl)	Men (%)	Women (%)
Diabetics		
Total	7.3	13.5
<35	10.3	37.5
35–44	13.2	10.3
45+	0.0	10.6
Non-diabetics		
Total	7.8	3.3
<35	10.8	9.1
35–44	10.1	4.7
45+	5.2	2.8

in women. Thus there was no lipid or lipoprotein abnormality that was associated with vascular disease in all groups of diabetics.

In a study of peripheral arteriosclerosis in diabetes[110] a significant negative correlation between HDL cholesterol and atherosclerosis was found in non-insulin-dependent diabetics treated by diet and also in non-insulin-dependent diabetics treated with insulin, but not in those treated with sulphonylureas or in insulin-dependent diabetics. LDL cholesterol was associated with atherosclerosis only in non-insulin-dependent diabetics treated with insulin, whereas VLDL triglyceride was significantly associated with atherosclerosis in insulin-treated diabetics whether NIDDM or IDDM. There was no statistical difference in the prevalence of arteriosclerosis in males and females in any of the treatment groups.

The evidence relating lipid abnormalities to large-vessel disease in diabetes is thus somewhat contradictory. However, it seems that in general, abnormalities in circulating lipids have the same relationship to atherosclerosis in diabetics as in non-diabetics, but do not entirely account for the association between diabetes and atherosclerosis.

CONCLUSIONS

A number of mechanisms produce disorders of lipid metabolism in diabetes. Depending on the type and severity of the diabetes, abnormal blood lipids may result from an increased supply of lipid substrate, enhanced synthesis of lipoproteins, or defective lipoprotein removal. Usually a number of mechanisms are operating at the same time. Although abnormal circulating lipid levels are relatively common in diabetics, they do not entirely explain the increased frequency of atherosclerosis in this condition.

References

1. Nikkila, F. A. (1973). Triglyceride metabolism in diabetes mellitus. *Progr. Biochem. Pharmacol.*, **8**, 271
2. Stout, R. W., Bierman, E. L. and Brunzell, J. D. (1975). Atherosclerosis and disorders of lipid metabolism in diabetes. In Vallance-Owen, J. (ed.) *Diabetes – its Physiological and Biochemical Basis*, pp. 125–69. (Lancaster: MTP Press)
3. Wilson, D. A. and Brown, W. V. (1978). Lipids and lipoproteins in diabetes mellitus. *Adv. Mod. Nutr.*, **2**, 127
4. Brunzell, J. D., Chait, A. and Bierman, E. L. (1978). Pathophysiology of lipoprotein transport. *Metabolism*, **27**, 1109
5. Bierman, E. L., Porte, D., Jr and Bagdade, J. D. (1970). Hypertriglyceridemia and glucose intolerance in man. In Jeanrenaud, B. and Hepp, D. (eds.) *Adipose Tissue*, pp. 209–12. (New York: Academic Press)
6. Bagdade, J. D., Bierman, E. L. and Porte, D. Jr. (1971). Influence of obesity on the relationship between insulin and triglyceride levels in endogenous hypertriglyceridemia. *Diabetes*, **20**, 664
7. Olefsky, J. M., Farquhar, J. W. and Reaven, G. M. (1974). Reappraisal of the role of insulin in hypertriglyceridemia. *Am. J. Med.*, **57**, 551
8. Brunzell, J. D. and Bierman, E. L. (1977). Plasma triglyceride and insulin levels in familial hypertriglyceridemia. *Ann. Intern. Med.*, **87**, 198
9. Kyner, J. L., Levy, R. I., Soeldner, J. S., Gleason, R. E. and Fredrickson, D. S. (1976). Lipid, glucose and insulin interrelationships in normal, prediabetic, and chemical diabetic subjects. *J. Lab. Clin. Med.*, **88**, 345
10. Tan, M. H., Havel, R. J., Gerich, J. E., Soeldner, J. S. and Kane, J. P. (1980). Pancreatic alpha and beta cell function in familial dysbetalipoproteinemia. *Horm. Metab. Res.*, **12**, 421
11. Topping, D. L. and Mayes, P. A. (1972). The immediate effects of insulin and fructose on the metabolism of the perfused liver: changes in lipoprotein secretion, fatty acid oxidation and esterification, lipogenesis and carbohydrate metabolism. *Biochem. J.*, **126**, 295

12. Reaven, E. P. and Reaven, G. M. (1974). Mechanisms for development of diabetic hypertriglyceridemia in streptozotocin-treated rats. Effect of diet and duration of insulin deficiency. *J. Clin. Invest.*, **54**, 1167
13. Balasse, E. O., Bier, D. M. and Havel, R. J. (1972). Early effects of anti-insulin serum on hepatic metabolism of plasma free fatty acids in dogs. *Diabetes*, **21**, 280
14. Renold, A. E., Crofford, O. B., Stauffacher, W. and Jeanrenaud, B. (1965). Hormonal control of adipose tissue metabolism, with special reference to the effects of insulin. *Diabetologia*, **1**, 4
15. Gross, R. C. and Carlson, L. A. (1968). Metabolic effects of nicotinic acid in acute insulin deficiency in the rat. *Diabetes*, **17**, 353
16. Bagdade, J. D., Porte, D. Jr. and Bierman, E. L. (1968). Acute insulin withdrawal and the regulation of plasma triglyceride removal in diabetic subjects. *Diabetes*, **17**, 127
17. Pykalisto, O. J., Smith, P. H. and Brunzell, J. D. (1975). Determinants of human adipose tissue lipoprotein lipase. Effect of diabetes and obesity on basal and diet-induced activity. *J. Clin. Invest.*, **56**, 1108
18. Chen, Y. I., Risser, T. R., Cully, M. and Reaven, G. M. (1979). Is the hyper-triglyceridemia associated with insulin deficiency caused by decreased lipoprotein lipase activity? *Diabetes*, **28**, 893
19. Greenfield, M., Kolterman, O., Olefsky, J. and Reaven, G. M. (1980). Mechanism of hypertriglyceridaemia in diabetic patients with fasting hyperglycaemia. *Diabetologia*, **18**, 441
20. Bagdade, J. D., Porte, D. Jr. and Bierman, E. L. (1967). Diabetic lipemia. A form of acquired fat-induced lipemia. *N. Engl. J. Med.*, **276**, 427
21. Brunzell, J. D., Porte, D. Jr. and Bierman, E. L. (1975). Reversible abnormalities in postheparin lipolytic activity during the late phase of release in diabetes mellitus (postheparin lipolytic activity in diabetes). *Metabolism*, **24**, 1123
22. Lewis, B., Mancini, M., Mattock, M., Chait, A. and Fraser, T. R. (1972). Plasma triglyceride and fatty acid metabolism in diabetes mellitus. *Eur. J. Clin. Invest.*, **2**, 445
23. Nikkila, E. A. and Kekki, M. (1973). Plasma triglyceride transport kinetics in diabetes mellitus. *Metabolism*, **22**, 1
24. Brunzell, J. D., Porte, D. Jr and Bierman, E. L. (1979). Abnormal lipoprotein-lipase-mediated plasma triglyceride removal in untreated diabetes mellitus associated with hypertriglyceridemia. *Metabolism*, **28**, 901
25. Taskinen, M.-R. and Nikkila, E. A. (1979). Lipoprotein lipase activity of adipose tissue and skeletal muscle in insulin-deficient human diabetes. *Diabetologia*, **17**, 351
26. Clarenburg, R. and Chaikoff, I. L. (1966). Cholesterol synthesis in liver of alloxan-diabetic rat: role of diet. *Am. J. Physiol.*, **210**, 37
27. Burns, B. J. and Elwood, J. C. (1969). Lipid metabolism in kidney and liver tissue from normal and diabetic rats. *Biochim. Biophys. Acta*, **187**, 307
28. Corder, C. N. and Kalkhoff, R. K. (1969). Hepatic lipid metabolism in alloxan diabetic rats. *J. Lab. Clin. Med.*, **73**, 551
29. Williams, W. R., Hill, R. and Chaikoff, I. L. (1960). Portal venous injection of insulin in the diabetic rat: time of induction of changes in hepatic lipogenesis, cholesterogenesis, and glycogenesis. *J. Lipid Res.*, **1**, 236
30. Stout, R. W. (1969). Insulin stimulation of cholesterol synthesis by arterial tissue. *Lancet*, **2**, 467
31. Stout, R. W. (1977). The effect of insulin and glucose on sterol synthesis in cultured rat arterial smooth muscle cells. *Atherosclerosis*, **27**, 271
32. Bathena, J., Avignan, J. and Schreiner, M. E. (1974). Effect of insulin on sterol and fatty acid synthesis and hydroxy methylglutaryl CoA reductase activity in mammalian cells grown in culture. *Proc. Natl. Acad. Sci., USA*, **71**, 2174
33. Lakshmanan, M. R., Nepokroeff, C. M., Ness, G. C., Dugan, R. E. and Porter, J. W. (1973). Stimulation by insulin of rat liver β-hydroxy β-methylglutaryl coenzyme A reductase and cholesterol synthesising activities. *Biochem. Biophys. Res. Commun.*, **50**, 704
34. Huber, J., Guder, W., Latzin, S. and Hamprecht, B. (1973). The influence of insulin and glucagon on hydroxy-methylglutaryl coenzyme A reductase activity in rat liver. *Hoppe-Seyler's Z. Physiol. Chem.*, **254**, 795

35. Nepokroeff, C. M., Lakshmanan, M. R., Ness, G. C., Dugan, R. E. and Porter, J. W. (1974). Regulation of the diurnal rhythm of rat liver β-methylglutaryl coenzyme A reductase activity by insulin, glucagon, cyclic AMP and hydrocortisone. *Arch. Biochem. Biophys.*, **160**, 387

36. Nakayama, H. and Nakagawa, S. (1977). Influence of streptozotocin diabetes on intestinal 3-hydroxy-3-methylglutaryl coenzyme A reductase activity in the rat. *Diabetes*, **26**, 439

37. Nervi, F. O., Genzalez, A. and Valdivieso, V. D. (1974). Studies on cholesterol metabolism in the diabetic rat. *Metabolism*, **23**, 495

38. Bennion, L. J. and Grundy, S. M. (1977). Effects of diabetes mellitus on cholesterol metabolism in man. *N. Engl. J. Med.*, **296**, 1365

39. Miettinen, T. A. (1971). Cholesterol production in obesity. *Circulation*, **44**, 842

40. Saudek, C. D. and Brach, E. L. (1978). Cholesterol metabolism in diabetes. *Diabetes*, **27**, 1059

41. Frier, B. M. and Saudek, C. D. (1979). Cholesterol metabolism in diabetes: the effect of insulin on the kinetics of plasma squalene. *J. Clin. Endocrinol. Metab.*, **49**, 824

42. Chait, A., Bierman, E. L. and Albers, J. J. (1978). Regulatory role of insulin in the degradation of low density lipoprotein by cultured human skin fibroblasts. *Biochim. Biophys. Acta*, **529**, 292

43. Chait, A., Bierman, E. L. and Albers, J. J. (1979). Low-density lipoprotein receptor activity in cultured human skin fibroblasts. Mechanisms of insulin-induced stimulation. *J. Clin. Invest.*, **64**, 1309

44. Chait, A., Bierman, E. L. and Albers, J. J. (1979). Low density lipoprotein receptor activity in fibroblasts cultured from diabetic donors. *Diabetes*, **28**, 914

45. Goldstein, J. L., Hazzard, W. R., Schrott, H. G., Bierman, E. L. and Motulsky, A. G. (1973). Hyperlipidemia in coronary heart disease. Lipid levels in 500 survivors of myocardial infarction. *J. Clin. Invest.*, **52**, 1533

46. Brunzell, J. D., Hazzard, W. R., Motulsky, A. G. and Bierman, E. L. (1975). Evidence for diabetes mellitus and genetic forms of hypertriglyceridemia as independent entities. *Metabolism*, **24**, 1115

47. Buchanan, K. D. (1977). Glucagon. In Bajaj, J. S. (ed.) *Insulin and Metabolism*, pp. 233–70. (Amsterdam, Elsevier/North Holland: Biomedical Press)

48. Lefebvre, P. (1975). Glucagon and adipose tissue. *Biochem. Pharmacol.*, **24**, 1261

49. Schade, D. S., Woodside, W. and Eaton, R. P. (1979). The role of glucagon in the regulation of plasma lipids. *Metabolism*, **28**, 874

50. Weinstein, I., Klausner, H. A. and Heimberg, M. (1973). The effect of concentration of glucagon on output of triglyceride, ketone bodies, glucose and urea by the liver. *Biochim. Biophys. Acta*, **296**, 300

51. Schweppe, J. S. and Jungmann, A. A. (1969). Effect of hormones on hepatic cholesterol ester synthesis *in vitro. Proc. Soc. Exp. Biol. Med.*, **131**, 868

52. Friedman, M., Byers, S. O., Rosenman, R. H. and Elel, S. (1971). Effect of glucagon on blood-cholesterol levels in rats. *Lancet*, **2**, 464

53. Caren, R. and Corbo, L. (1960). Glucagon and cholesterol metabolism. *Metabolism*, **9**, 938

54. Hoak, J. C., Connor, W. E. and Warner, E. D. (1968). Toxic effects of glucagon-induced acute lipid mobilisation in geese. *J. Clin. Invest.*, **47**, 2701

55. Grande, F. and Prigge, W. F. (1970). Glucagon infusion, plasma FFA and triglycerides, blood sugar and liver lipids in birds. *Am. J. Physiol.*, **218**, 1406

56. Caren, R. and Corbo, L. (1971). Depression of plasma lipid fractions and inhibition of platelet aggregation by action of glucagon. *Metabolism*, **20**, 1057

57. Amatuzio, D. S., Grande, F. and Wada, S. (1962). Effect of glucagon on the serum lipids in essential hyperlipemia and in hypercholesterolemia. *Metabolism*, **11**, 1240

58. Caren, R. and Corbo, L. (1974). Glucagon and plasma lipoprotein lipase. *Proc. Soc. Exp. Biol. Med.*, **146**, 1106

59. Schade, D. S. and Eaton, R. P. (1975). Modulation of fatty acid metabolism by glucagon in man. III. Role of pharmacologic limitation of FFA availability. *Diabetes*, **24**, 1020

60. Marks, V., Frizel, D., Twycross, R. G. and Buchanan, K. D. (1971). Effect of β-pyridylcarbinol on glucose tolerance, plasma glucagon, insulin and growth hormone in

man. In Grey, K. F. and Carlson, L. A. (eds.) *Metabolic Effect of Nicotinic Acid and Derivatives*, pp. 961–75. (Berne: Huber)

61. Tiengo, A., Muggeo, M., Assan, R., Fedele, D. and Crepaldi, G. (1975). Glucagon secretion in primary endogenous hypertriglyceridemia before and after clofibrate treatment. *Metabolism*, **24**, 901

62. Eaton, R. P. and Schade, D. S. (1973). Glucagon resistance as a hormonal basis for endogenous hyperlipaemia. *Lancet*, **1**, 973

63. Schade, D. S. and Eaton, R. P. (1977). The effect of short term physiological elevations of plasma glucagon concentration on plasma triglyceride concentration in normal and diabetic man. *Horm. Metab. Res.*, **9**, 253

64. Kaufmann, R. L., Assal, J. P., Soeldner, J. S., Wilmshurst, E. G., Lemaire, J. R., Gleason, R. E. and White, P. (1975). Plasma lipid levels in diabetic children. Effect of diet restricted in cholesterol and saturated fats. *Diabetes*, **24**, 672

65. Chase, H. P. and Glasgow, A. M. (1976). Juvenile diabetes mellitus and serum lipids and lipoprotein levels. *Am. J. Dis. Child.*, **130**, 1113

66. Chance, G. W., Albutt, E. C. and Edkins, S. M. (1969). Serum lipids and lipoproteins in untreated diabetic children. *Lancet*, **1**, 1126

67. Wilson, D. E., Schreibman, P. H., Day, V. C. and Arky, R. A. (1970). Hyperlipidemia in an adult diabetic population. *J. Chron. Dis.*, **23**, 501

68. Hayes, T. M. (1972). Plasma lipoproteins in adult diabetes. *Clin. Endocrinol.*, **1**, 247

69. Rodger, N. W. and Du, E. L. (1973). Some factors indicative of hypertriglyceridemia in patients investigated for diabetes mellitus. *Can. Med. Assoc. J.*, **109**, 363

70. Schonfeld, G., Birge, C., Miller, J. P., Kessler, G. and Santiago, J. (1974). Apolipoprotein composition in diabetes. *Diabetes*, **23**, 827

71. Miller, G. J. and Miller, N. E. (1975). Plasma high-density lipoprotein concentration and the development of ischaemic heart disease. *Lancet*, **1**, 16

72. Gordon, T., Castelli, W. P., Hjortland, M. C., Kannel, W. B. and Dawber, T. R. (1977). High density lipoprotein as a protective factor against coronary heart disease. *Am. J. Med.*, **62**, 707

73. Rossner, S., Kjellin, K. G., Mettinger, K. L., Siden, A. and Soderstrom, C. E. (1978). Normal serum-cholesterol but low HDL-cholesterol concentration in young patients with ischaemic cerebrovascular disease. *Lancet*, **1**, 577

74. Taggart, H. and Stout, R. W. (1979). Reduced high density lipoprotein in stroke: relationship with elevated triglyceride and hypertension. *Eur. J. Clin. Invest.*, **9**, 219

75. Lopes-Virella, M. F. L., Stone, P. G. and Colwell, J. A. (1977). Serum high density lipoprotein in diabetic patients. *Diabetologia*, **13**, 285

76. Paisey, R., Elkeles, R. S., Hambley, J. and Magill, P. (1978). The effects of chlorpropamide and insulin on serum lipids lipoproteins and fractional triglyceride removal. *Diabetologia*, **15**, 81

77. Kennedy, A. L., Lappin, T. R. J., Lavery, T. D., Hadden, D. R., Weaver, J. A. and Montgomery, D.A.D. (1978). Relation of high-density lipoprotein cholesterol concentration to type of diabetes and its control. *Br. Med. J.*, **2**, 1191

78. Calvert, G. D., Graham, J. J., Mannik, T., Wise, P. H. and Yeates, R. A. (1978). Effects of therapy on plasma-high-density-lipoprotein-cholesterol concentration in diabetes mellitus. *Lancet*, **2**, 66

79. Howard, B. V., Savage, P. J., Bennion, L. J. and Bennett, P. H. (1978). Lipoprotein composition in diabetes mellitus. *Atherosclerosis*, **30**, 153

80. Nikkila, E. A. and Hormila, P. (1978). Serum lipids and lipoproteins in insulin-treated diabetes. *Diabetes*, **27**, 1078

81. Elkeles, R. S., Wu, J. and Hambley, J. (1978). Haemoglobin A, blood glucose and high-density lipoprotein cholesterol in insulin-requiring diabetes. *Lancet*, **2**, 547

82. Gordon, T., Castelli, W. P., Hjortland, M. C., Kannel, W. B. and Dawber, T. R. (1977). Diabetes, blood lipids, and the role of obesity in coronary heart disease risk for women. The Framingham Study. *Ann. Intern. Med.*, **87**, 393

83. Eckel, R. H., Albers, J. J., Cheung, M. C., Wahl, P. W., Lindgren, F. T. and Bierman, E. L. (1981). High density lipoprotein composition in insulin dependent diabetes mellitus. *Diabetes*, **30**, 132

84. Olefsky, J., Reaven, G. M. and Farquhar, J. W. (1974). Effects of weight reduction on

obesity. Studies of lipid and carbohydrate metabolism in normal and hyperlipoproteinemic subjects. *J. Clin. Invest.*, **53**, 64
85. Stout, R. W., Brunzell, J. D., Porte, D. Jr and Bierman, E. L. (1974). Effect of phenformin on lipid transport in hypertriglyceridemia. *Metabolism*, **23**, 815
86. Stone, D. B. and Connor, W. E. (1963). The prolonged effects of a low cholesterol, high carbohydrate diet upon the serum lipids in diabetic patients. *Diabetes*, **12**, 127
87. Sterky, G. C. G., Persson, B. E. H. and Larsson, Y. A. A. (1966). Dietary fats, the diurnal blood lipids and ketones in juvenile diabetes. *Diabetologia*, **2**, 14
88. Hockaday, T. D. R., Hockaday, J. M., Mann, J. I. and Turner, R. C. (1978). Prospective comparison of modified fat high carbohydrate with standard low carbohydrate dietary advice in the treatment of diabetes: one year follow-up study. *Br. J. Nutr.*, **39**, 357
89. Brunzell, J. D., Lerner, R. L., Hazzard, W. R., Porte, D. Jr and Bierman, E. L. (1971). Improved glucose tolerance with high carbohydrate feeding in mild diabetes. *N. Engl. J. Med.*, **284**, 521
90. Brunzell, J. D., Lerner, R. L., Porte, D., Jr and Bierman, E. L. (1974). Effect of a fat-free, high carbohydrate diet on diabetic subjects with fasting hyperglycemia. *Diabetes*, **23**, 138
91. Weinsier, R. L., Seeman, A., Herrera, G. M., Assal, J. P., Soeldner, J. S. and Gleason, R. E. (1974). High- and low-carbohydrate diets in diabetes mellitus. Study of effects on diabetic control, insulin secretion and blood lipids. *Ann. Intern. Med.*, **80**, 332
92. Perrett, A. D., Rowe, A. S., Shahmanesh, M., Allison, S. P. and Hartog, M. (1974). Blood lipids in treated diabetics. *Diabetologia*, **10**, 115
93. Simpson, R. W., Mann, J. I., Hockaday, T. D. R., Hockaday, J. M., Turner, R. C. and Jefls, R. (1979). Lipid abnormalities in untreated maturity-onset diabetics and the effect of treatment. *Diabetologia*, **16**, 101
94. Dunn, F. L., Pietri, A. and Raskin, P. (1981). Plasma lipid and lipoprotein levels with continuous subcutaneous insulin infusion in type 1 diabetes mellitus. *Ann. Intern. Med.*, **95**, 426
95. Lisch, H. J. and Sailer, S. (1981). Lipoprotein patterns in diet, sulphonylurea and insulin treated diabetics. *Diabetologia*, **20**, 118
96. Lopes-Virella, M. F., Wohltmann, H. J., Loadholt, C. B. and Buse, M. G. (1981). Plasma lipids and lipoproteins in young insulin-dependent diabetic patients: relationship with control. *Diabetologia*, **21**, 216
97. Sosenko, J. M., Breslow, J. L., Miettinen, O. S. and Gabbay, K. H. (1980). Hyperglycemia and plasma lipid levels. A prospective study of young insulin-dependent diabetic patients. *N. Engl. J. Med.*, **302**, 650
98. Albrink, M. J., Lavietes, P. H. and Man, E. B. (1962). Relationship between serum lipids and the vascular complications of diabetes from 1931 to 1961. *Trans. Assoc. Am. Phys.*, **75**, 235
99. Reinheimer, W., Bliffen, G., McCoy, J., Wallace, D. and Albrink, M. J. (1967). Weight gain, serum lipids and vascular disease in diabetics. *Am. J. Clin. Nutr.*, **20**, 986
100. New, M. I., Roberts, T. N., Bierman, E. L. and Reader, G. G. (1963). The significance of blood lipid alterations in diabetes mellitus. *Diabetes*, **12**, 208
101. Kudo, H. (1969). Serum triglyceride levels of untreated diabetics in relation to vascular lesions and obesity. *Tohoku J. Exp. Med.*, **97**, 47
102. Santen, R. J., Willis, P. W. and Fajans, S. S. (1972). Atherosclerosis in diabetes mellitus. *Arch. Intern. Med.*, **130**, 833
103. Ostrander, L. D., Neff, B. J., Block, W. D., Francis, T. and Epstein, F. H. (1967). Hyperglycemia and hypertriglyceridemia among persons with coronary heart disease. *Ann. Intern. Med.*, **67**, 34
104. Ostrander, L. D., Lamphiear, D. E., Carman, W. J. and Williams, G. W. (1981). Blood glucose and risk of coronary disease. *Arteriosclerosis*, **1**, 33
105. Fuller, J. H., Shipley, M. J., Rose, G., Jarrett, R. J. and Keen, H. (1980). Coronary-heart-disease risk and impaired glucose tolerance. *Lancet*, **1**, 1373
106. Garcia, M. J., McNamara, P. M., Gordon, T. and Kannel, W. B. (1974). Morbidity and mortality in diabetics in the Framingham population. Sixteen year follow-up study. *Diabetes*, **23**, 105
107. Kannel, W. B. and McGee, D. L. (1979). Diabetes and cardiovascular risk factors: the

Framingham Study. *Circulation*, **59**, 8
108. Kannel, W. B. and McGee, D. L. (1979). Diabetes and glucose tolerance as risk factors for cardiovascular disease: the Framingham Study. *Diabetes Care*, **2**, 120
109. Reckless, J. P. D., Betteridge, D. J., Wu, P., Payne, B. and Galton, D. J. (1978). High-density and low-density lipoproteins and prevalence of vascular disease in diabetes mellitus. *Br. Med. J.*, **1**, 883
110. Beach, K. W., Brunzell, J. D., Conquest, L. L. and Strandness, D. E. (1979). The correlation of arteriosclerosis obliterans with lipoproteins in insulin-dependent and non-insulin-dependent diabetes. *Diabetes*, **28**, 836

6
Insulin and atherosclerosis

This chapter will discuss clinical and epidemiological evidence that elevated insulin levels are associated with atherosclerosis and its complications. Evidence that insulin has biological actions on the arterial wall which may be relevant to the development of atheromatous lesions is discussed in Chapter 7.

DIABETES MELLITUS

Although relative or absolute insulin deficiency is the cause of abnormal glucose tolerance, the tissues of the diabetic may be exposed to high concentrations of insulin. The reasons for this differ in non-insulin-dependent and insulin-dependent diabetics.

Insulin is secreted from at least two functional pools, one of which, the slowly releasable synthesis-dependent pool, is mainly responsible for basal insulin secretion, while the rapidly releasable storage pool is responsible for the acute insulin response to glucose stimulation[1]. In normal subjects, basal and stimulated insulin levels are linearly related, and there is also a linear relationship between relative body weight and basal insulin secretion[2]. In diabetics the relationship between basal insulin and obesity is unaltered[1]. Even when ketotic, diabetics have normal basal insulin levels. However, the acute insulin response to glucose is impaired in diabetics, whether the glucose is given orally or intravenously. Thus, if weight-matched diabetics and non-diabetics are compared, they will have equal basal insulin levels but the diabetics will have a lower insulin response to glucose. Non-insulin-dependent diabetics are frequently obese[3]. As obesity is associated with elevations of both fasting and post-glucose insulin levels irrespective of the presence of diabetes, non-insulin-dependent diabetics who are obese will have higher insulin levels than non-diabetics who are thin. In addition, mild diabetes of the type which is commonly associated with an increased incidence of atherosclerosis is also associated with high insulin levels[4-7].

The majority of studies of atherosclerosis in diabetes have not taken into account the weight of the diabetics and the non-diabetic controls. However, two studies have shown that the large-vessel complications of diabetes are associated with excessive weight gain or obesity[8,9].

Insulin-dependent diabetics with fasting hyperglycaemia and a tendency to ketoacidosis have an absolute deficiency of insulin and are treated with insulin. The dose of insulin administered to diabetics is considerably greater than the 20–30 units which is the normal daily output of the pancreatic islets[10]. Furthermore, the regulation of insulin in relation to blood glucose levels and nutrient intake in insulin-treated diabetics is abnormal. Insulin is absorbed from the injection site at a rate which is unrelated to meals or blood glucose levels, and at times during the day circulating insulin levels will be higher in the insulin-treated diabetic than in the non-diabetic[11]. In the non-diabetic insulin is secreted directly into the portal vein where it has its major activity on the liver. 50% of secreted insulin is removed on first passage through the liver and insulin levels in the portal vein are much higher than those in the peripheral circulation[12]. In the diabetic treated with insulin, abnormally high concentrations of insulin have to be achieved in the systemic circulation in order to achieve adequate concentrations in the liver. For all these reasons, insulin levels in insulin-treated diabetics may be abnormally high. Long-term treatment with insulin induces the formation of insulin antibodies, which bind and probably inactivate some of the insulin, resulting in an increase in the patient's insulin requirements[13]. A number of studies of insulin levels in insulin-treated diabetics have been reported and the results have been contradictory. Some studies have shown fasting insulin levels that are normal or elevated, sometimes grossly, in insulin-treated diabetics 14–24 h after their last insulin injection[14–17]. Other workers have shown abnormally low fasting free insulin levels in insulin-treated diabetics[18]. Clearly the technical problems in the measurements have to be resolved before firm conclusions can be drawn on the insulin levels in insulin-treated diabetics.

Thus whether because of therapy or because of coexisting obesity, few diabetics are truly insulin-deficient, and many diabetics appear to have excessive levels of circulating insulin.

There have been only two studies of the relationship of atherosclerosis in diabetes to circulating insulin levels. When diabetics with ischaemic heart disease were compared with subjects with diabetes and no evidence of ischaemic heart disease[19], oral glucose tolerance was the same in the two groups, but the atherosclerotic subjects had slightly higher insulin responses to oral glucose, and higher peak insulin responses to oral tolbutamide. In patients not receiving insulin therapy, the ratios of insulin to glucose were significantly higher in the diabetics with atherosclerosis[9]. There is thus some evidence to suggest that elevated insulin levels may be associated with atherosclerosis in diabetics not receiving insulin therapy. However, the numbers studied have been small and the evidence is still fairly weak.

ATHEROSCLEROSIS IN NON-DIABETICS

Because of the frequent finding of abnormal glucose tolerance in patients with ischaemic vascular disease, insulin levels during glucose tolerance tests have been measured in patients with atherosclerosis. Subjects with disease of coronary arteries[19-27], cerebral arteries[28] and the arteries of the lower limbs[27,29,30] have elevated insulin responses to oral glucose compared to control subjects without evidence of vascular disease. The studies differ in a number of ways and provide answers to different questions.

The cause of the abnormal insulin response

Insulin responses to intravenous glucose[19] or to intravenous tolbutamide[22,24] have been less clearly elevated than responses to oral glucose in atherosclerotic subjects, suggesting that a gastrointestinal factor might be involved in the high insulin response to oral glucose.

Insulin levels in arterial disease without ischaemia

Atherosclerosis is usually diagnosed by the presence of ischaemia or infarction in the organ supplied by the affected artery. However, two studies have used angiographic evidence of coronary[23] or peripheral[29] arterial disease and have shown that elevated insulin responses are present in the absence of complete occlusion and infarction. In contrast, in the acute phase of myocardial infarction and in congestive cardiac failure, depression of the insulin response to oral glucose is found[31], perhaps due to overactivity of the sympathetic nervous system. It appears therefore that high insulin levels are associated with the arterial disease itself.

The relationship of insulin to other risk factors for atherosclerosis

Hypertriglyceridaemia is associated with atherosclerosis in diabetics[9,32], and in non-diabetics it is an important risk factor for ischaemic heart disease[33]. A number of studies have reported a significant correlation between insulin levels and triglyceride levels in normal and hypertriglyceridaemic non-diabetic subjects[34,35]. The role of insulin in triglyceride metabolism is complex and somewhat contradictory. Insulin can directly stimulate triglyceride production in the liver[36]. Insulin is also necessary for the full activity of the lipoprotein lipase enzyme system[37] and inhibits adipose tissue lipase[38] reducing the supply of free fatty acid substrate for triglyceride synthesis. Thus, changes in insulin secretion can alter triglyceride levels in several different ways.

It has been known for many years that morbidity and mortality are higher among the overweight than those whose weight is normal[39]. Obesity is associated with increased circulating insulin levels. There is a direct correlation between obesity and basal insulin secretion[2] and this is maintained in diabetes. In non-diabetic subjects there is also a positive relationship between the magnitude of the insulin response to glucose and the basal insulin level[2]. Thus obese subjects, both diabetic and non-diabetic, have higher circulating insulin levels than thin subjects.

Patients with chronic renal failure have a high incidence of premature and extensive atherosclerosis[40]. Although hypertension is often present in chronic renal failure and may contribute to atherosclerosis, disorders of carbohydrate and lipid metabolism also occur. Carbohydrate intolerance has been a well-recognized feature of uraemia for many years[41]. Elevated basal insulin concentrations are also found[42] and the insulin response to various stimuli, expressed in terms of basal insulin, is deficient in uraemic subjects[41]. Following intensive haemodialysis, basal insulin levels fall.

In investigations that have included other risk factors for atherosclerosis, including blood pressure and serum cholesterol[23,29] it has been found that the relationship of elevated insulin levels to arterial disease is independent of the influence of serum lipids or blood pressure. In three prospective studies multivariate analysis showed that the risk associated with elevated insulin levels was independent of other risk factors including cholesterol, blood pressure and blood sugar.

Insulin levels in populations with different incidences of atherosclerosis

In South Africa the white population has a much higher incidence of ischaemic heart disease than the Bantu population. Insulin responses to glucose in the white population are almost twice as high as those in the Bantu population[43]. Edinburgh men have a higher incidence of ischaemic heart disease than men in Stockholm. Although the glucose responses to oral glucose were identical in Edinburgh and Stockholm, the insulin responses to oral glucose were significantly higher in the Scottish men than in the Swedish men[44]. Edinburgh and Stockholm also differed in other risk factors for atherosclerosis, including blood pressure and serum lipids.

Prospective studies of insulin in relation to coronary heart disease

Three prospective studies of the relationship of insulin levels to ischaemic heart disease have been carried out (Table 6.1). In the Helsinki Policemen study[45] elevated fasting and post-glucose plasma insulin levels had a strong predictive value for the development of coronary artery disease over a 5-year period. Multivariate analysis showed that the predictive value of plasma insulin responses to oral glucose was independent of other risk factors including plasma cholesterol, blood pressure and blood glucose. In the Paris study[46] elevated plasma insulin levels and insulin : glucose ratios were associated with an increased risk of coronary artery disease and the association was independent of other risk factors. In Busselton, Australia, there was positive relationship between insulin responses 1 h after glucose and the incidence of and mortality from coronary heart disease in men aged 60–69[47]. The relationship was also present in all men and was independent of other major risk factors. This association was not found in women. These studies provide the first evidence of the predictive value of raised plasma insulin levels in the development of ischaemic heart disease.

CONCLUSIONS

The clinical and epidemiological evidence linking high insulin levels with atherosclerosis is both circumstantial and direct. Particularly impressive are

Table 6.1 Prospective studies of insulin and cardiovascular disease

	Busselton, Australia[47]	Helsinki, Finland[45]	Paris, France[46]
Sex	men and women	men	men
Age	<40–70+	30–59	43–54
Blood sampling for insulin	1 h after 50 g glucose (non-fasting)	Fasting 1 h, 2 h after 75 g or 90 g glucose	Fasting 2 h after 75 g glucose
End-point	6 year incidence 12 year mortality	MI CHD death; other CHD (5-year)	MI CHD death (63 months)
Other risk factors	blood pressure blood sugar cholesterol uric acid	blood pressure blood sugar body mass index cholesterol triglyceride smoking	blood pressure blood sugar body mass index cholesterol triglyceride smoking
Relation to CHD	1 h insulin in men aged 60+	fasting, 1 h, 2 h and sum insulin in whole group	fasting and 2 h insulin and insulin : glucose ratio in whole group

CHD = Coronary heart disease; MI = myocardial infarction

the results of three prospective studies all indicating a predictive role of insulin in ischaemic heart disease. The design and results of the three studies differed, and further investigation is necessary to confirm or refute some of the results, particularly with respect to the effects of age and sex. Similar prospective studies on the predictive role of insulin in atherosclerosis in diabetics are urgently required. Such studies would present no technical problems in non-insulin-dependent diabetics but measurement of plasma insulin is difficult in insulin-treated diabetics. At present there are only the results of two small cross-sectional studies of insulin in relation to atherosclerosis in diabetics. The results are consistent with the findings of the prospective studies in non-diabetics. High levels of circulating insulin are common in diabetics and the possibility of an association between this and the high incidence of atherosclerosis is worthy of consideration.

As discussed in detail in the next chapter, insulin has biological actions on the arterial wall which might be related to the pathogenesis of atherosclerosis. Based on the clinical epidemiological and experimental evidence, a hypothesis has been presented linking insulin with atherosclerosis[20,48,49] (Figure 6.1). This suggests that a primary abnormality is increased secretion of insulin and that atherosclerosis and some of its metabolic accompaniments are directly related to the effect of increased circulating insulin levels.

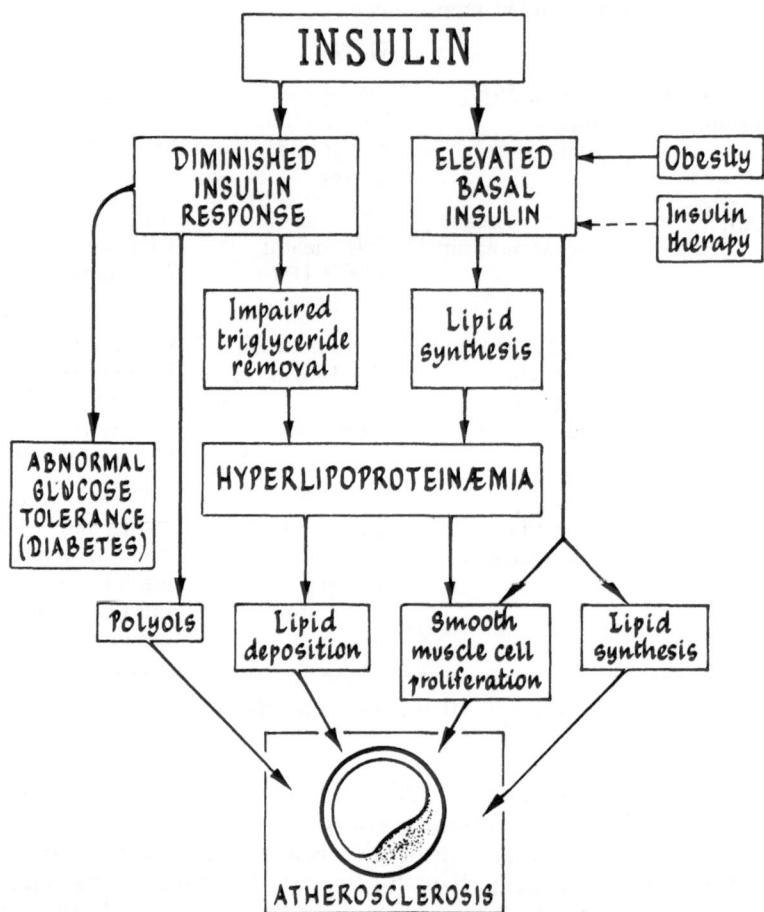

Figure 6.1 Scheme linking abnormal insulin levels to atherosclerosis and its accompanying disorders of lipid and carbohydrate metabolism[49]

References

1. Porte, D., Jr and Bagdade, J. (1970). Human insulin secretion: an integrated approach. *Annu. Rev. Med.*, **21**, 219
2. Bagdade, J. D., Bierman, E. L. and Porte, D., Jr (1967). The significance of basal insulin levels in evaluation of the insulin response to glucose in diabetic and non-diabetic subjects. *J. Clin. Invest.*, **46**, 1549
3. Pyke, D. A. and Please, N. W. (1957). Obesity, parity and diabetes. *J. Endocrinol.*, **15**, xxvi

4. Danowski, T. S., Lombardo, Y. B., Mendelsohn, L. V., Corredor, D. G., Morgan, C. R. and Sabeh, G. (1969). Insulin patterns prior to and after onset of diabetes. *Metabolism*, **18**, 731

5. Jackson, W. P. U., van Mieghem, W. and Keller, P. (1972). Insulin excess as the initial lesion in diabetes. *Lancet*, **1**, 1040

6. Reaven, G. M., Olefsky, J. and Farquhar, J. W. (1972). Does hyperglycaemia or hyperinsulinaemia characterise the patient with chemical diabetes. *Lancet*, **1**, 1247

7. Savage, P. J., Dippe, S. E., Bennett, P. H., Gordon, P., Roth, J., Rushforth, N. B. and Miller, M. (1975). Hyperinsulinemia and hypoinsulinemia. Insulin reponses to oral carbohydrate over a wide spectrum of glucose tolerance. *Diabetes*, **24**, 363

8. Reinheimer, W., Bliffen, G., McCoy, J., Wallace, D. and Albrink, M.J. (1967). Weight gain, serum lipids, and vascular disease in diabetics. *Am. J. Clin. Nutr.*, **20**, 986

9. Santen, R. J., Willis, P. W. and Fajans, S. S. (1972). Atherosclerosis in diabetes mellitus. *Arch. Intern. Med.*, **130**, 833

10. Goodner, C. J. and Porte, D., Jr (1972). Determinants of basal insulin secretion in man. In *Handbook of Physiology*. Section 7, Part 1, pp. 597–609. (Washington, DC: American Physiological Society)

11. Werther, G. A., Jenkins, P. A., Turner, R. C. and Baum, J. D. (1980). Twenty-four-hour metabolic profiles in diabetic children receiving insulin injections once or twice daily. *Br. Med. J.*, **2**, 414

12. Blackard, W. G. and Nelson, N. C. (1970). Portal and peripheral vein immunoreactive insulin concentrations before and after glucose infusion. *Diabetes*, **19**, 302

13. Rasmussen, S. M., Heding, I. G. and Parbst, E. (1975). Serum IRI in insulin-treated diabetics during a 24-hour period. *Diabetologia*, **11**, 151

14. Grodsky, G. M. (1965). Production of autoantibodies to insulin in man and rabbits. *Diabetes*, **14**, 396

15. Pearson, M. J. and Martin, F. I. R. (1970). The separation of total plasma insulin from binding proteins using gel filtration: its application to the measurement of rate of insulin disappearance. *Diabetologia*, **6**, 581

16. Heding, L. G. (1972). Determination of total serum insulin (IRI) in insulin-treated diabetic patients. *Diabetologia*, **8**, 260

17. Gennaro, W. D. and Van Norman, J. D. (1975). Quantitation of free, total and antibody-bound insulin in insulin-treated diabetics. *Clin. Chem.*, **21**, 873

18. Nakagawa, S., Nakayama, H., Sasaki, T., Yoshino, K., Yu, Y. Y., Shinozaki, K., Aoki, S. and Mashimo, K. (1973). A simple method for the determination of serum free insulin levels in insulin-treated patients. *Diabetes*, **22**, 590

19. Kashyap, L., Magill, F., Rojes, L. and Hoffman, M. M. (1970). Insulin and non-esterified fatty acid metabolism in asymptomatic diabetics and atherosclerotic subjects. *Can. Med. Assoc. J.*, **102**, 1165

20. Stout, R. W. (1977). The relationship of abnormal circulating insulin levels to atherosclerosis. *Atherosclerosis*, **27**, 1

21. Peters, N. and Hales, C. N. (1965). Plasma insulin concentrations after myocardial infarction. *Lancet*, **1**, 1144

22. Nikkila, E. A., Miettinen, A. A., Vesenne, M. R. and Pelkonen, R. (1965). Plasma insulin in coronary heart disease. *Lancet*, **2**, 508

23. Tzagournis, M., Chiles, R., Ryan, J. M. and Skillman, T. G. (1968). Interrelationships of hyperinsulinism and hypertriglyceridemia in young patients in coronary heart disease. *Circulation*, **38**, 1156

24. Christiansen, I., Derkert, T., Kjerulf, K., Mitgaard, K. and Worning, H. (1968). Glucose tolerance, plasma lipids and serum insulin in patients with ischaemic heart disease. *Acta Med. Scand.*, **184**, 283

25. Malherbe, C., De Gasparo, M., Berthet, P., De Hertogh, R. and Hoet, J. J. (1970). The pattern of plasma insulin response to glucose in patients with a previous myocardial infarction – the respective effects of age and disease. *Eur. J. Clin. Invest.*, **1**, 265

26. Gertler, M. M., Leetma, H. E., Saluste, E., Rosenberger, J. L. and Guthrie, R. G. (1972). Ischaemic heart disease – insulin, carbohydrate and lipid interrelationships. *Circulation*, **46**, 103

27. Sorge, F., Schwartzkopff, W. and Neuhaus, G. A. (1976). Insulin response to oral glucose

in patients with a previous myocardial infarction and in patients with peripheral vascular disease. *Diabetes*, **25**, 586

28. Gertler, M. M., Leetma, H. E., Saluste, E., Covalt, D. A. and Rosenberger, J. L. (1972). Covert diabetes mellitus ischaemic heart and cerebrovascular disease. *Geriatrics*, **27**, 105

29. Sloan, J. M., Mackay, J. S. and Sheridan, B. (1971). The incidence of plasma insulin, blood sugar and serum lipid abnormalities in patients with atherosclerotic disease. *Diabetologia*, **7**, 431

30. Welborn, T. A., Breckenbridge, A., Rubenstein, A. H., Dollery, C. T. and Fraser, T. R. (1966). Serum-insulin in essential hypertension and peripheral vascular disease. *Lancet*, **1**, 1336

31. Taylor, S. H. and Majid, P. A. (1971). Insulin and the heart. *J. Molec. Cell. Cardiol.*, **2**, 293

32. Ostrander, L. D., Neff, B. J., Block, W. D., Francis, T. and Epstein, F. H. (1967). Hyperglycemia and hypertriglyceridemia among persons with coronary heart disease. *Ann. Intern. Med.*, **67**, 34

33. Carlson, L. A. and Bottiger, O. E. (1972). Ischaemic heart disease in relation to fasting values of plasma triglycerides and cholesterol. *Lancet*, **1**, 865

34. Bierman, E. L., Porte, D., Jr and Bagdade, J. D. (1970). Hypertriglyceridemia and glucose intolerance in man. In Jeanrenaud, B. and Hepp, D. (eds.) *Adipose Tissue*, pp. 209–12. (New York: Academic Press)

35. Olefsky, J. M., Farquhar, J. W. and Reaven, G. M. (1974). Reappraisal of the role of insulin in hypertriglyceridemia. *Am. J. Med.*, **57**, 551

36. Topping, D. L. and Mayes, P. A. (1972). The immediate effects of insulin and fructose on the metabolism of the perfused liver – changes in lipoprotein secretion, fatty acid oxidation and esterification, lipogenesis and carbohydrate metabolism. *Biochem. J.*, **126**, 295

37. Bagdade, J. D., Porte, D., Jr and Bierman, E. L. (1968). Acute insulin withdrawal and the regulation of plasma triglyceride removal in diabetic subjects. *Diabetes*, **17**, 127

38. Renold, A. E., Crofford, O. B., Stauffacher, W. and Jeanrenaud, B. (1965). Hormonal control of adipose tissue metabolism, with special reference to the effects of insulin. *Diabetologia*, **1**, 4

39. Society of Actuaries (1959). *Build and Blood Pressure Study*. (Chicago: Society of Actuaries)

40. Lindner, A., Charra, B., Sherrard, D. J. and Scribner, B. H. (1974). Accelerated atherosclerosis in prolonged maintenance hemodialysis. *N. Engl. J. Med.*, **290**, 697

41. Bagdade, J. D. (1975). Disorders of carbohydrate and lipid metabolism in uremia. *Nephron*, **14**, 153

42. Bagdade, J. D. (1970). Uremic lipemia. *Arch. Intern. Med.*, **126**, 875

43. Rubenstein, A. H., Seftel, H. C., Miller, K., Bersohn, I. and Wright, A. D. (1969). Metabolic responses to oral glucose in healthy South African white, Indian and African subjects. *Br. Med. J.*, **1**, 748

44. Logan, R. L., Thomson, M., Riemersma, R. A., Oliver, M. F., Olsson, A. G., Rossner, S., Callmer, E., Walldius, G., Kaijser, L., Carlson, L. A., Lockerbie, L. and Lutz, W. (1978). Risk factors for ischaemic heart disease in normal men aged 40 (Edinburgh–Stockholm Study). *Lancet*, **1**, 949

45. Pyorala, K. (1979). Relationship of glucose tolerance and plasma insulin to the incidence of coronary heart disease: results from two population studies in Finland. *Diabetes Care*, **2**, 131

46. Ducimetiere, P., Eschwege, L., Papoz, J. L., Claude, R. J. R. and Rosselin, G. (1980). Relationship of plasma insulin levels to the incidence of myocardial infarction and coronary heart disease mortality in a middle-aged population. *Diabetologia*, **19**, 205

47. Welborn, T. A. and Wearne, K. (1979). Coronary heart disease incidence and cardiovascular mortality in Busselton with reference to glucose and insulin concentrations. *Diabetes Care*, **2**, 154

48. Stout, R. W. and Vallance-Owen, J. (1969). Insulin and atheroma. *Lancet*, **1**, 1078

49. Stout, R. W. (1979). Diabetes and atherosclerosis – the role of insulin. *Diabetologia*, **16**, 141

7
Vascular disease and experimental diabetes

EXPERIMENTAL VASCULAR DISEASE

Although the production of arterial lesions in animals fed high fat and cholesterol diets had been described at the beginning of the twentieth century, and experimental models of diabetes were available at the time Banting and Best isolated insulin in 1920, it was not until the 1940s that attempts were made to study the interaction of diabetes and atherosclerosis in the experimental animal. The first report of vascular lesions in an animal with experimental diabetes was that of Dragstedt and colleagues in 1940[1]. They noted that dogs which were pancreatectomized and kept alive with insulin injections had an abnormally high frequency of lipid-containing lesions in their aortas compared to control dogs.

The first systematic studies of atherosclerosis in animals with experimental diabetes were reported simultaneously in 1949[2,3]. The experimental design and results of these two studies were very similar. Rabbits were made diabetic with alloxan and fed high-cholesterol diets. After 50–90 days the aortas were examined for the presence of lesions. In both studies it was found that despite higher cholesterol levels the diabetic animals developed considerably less atherosclerosis than the controls (Table 7.1). This result was described as 'unexpected' by one group[2] and 'astonishing' by the other[3]. The possibility that alloxan was responsible for the apparently paradoxical result was rejected because some animals which had been given alloxan had transiently developed diabetes but then recovered again, and the aortas of these animals had the same degree of atherosclerosis as the controls. The possibility that the alloxan-recovered animals were constitutionally different from the other animals was ruled out by a later study[4] in which the pancreas was isolated from the circulation at the time the alloxan was administered. In this way the animals were exposed to alloxan but diabetes was not produced. The alloxan diabetic animals had higher serum cholesterol levels but less atherosclerosis than the controls, but the alloxan-treated animals whose pancreas had been protected had similar vascular lesions to the non-diabetic controls (Table

Table 7.1 Effect of alloxan diabetes on experimental atherosclerosis in the cholesterol-fed rabbit

	Blood glucose (mg/dl)	Serum cholesterol (mg/dl)	Atherosclerosis grade
Control	121	346	1.77
Diabetic	433	399	0.44
Alloxan recovered	122	389	2.6

Average figures calculated from Duff and McMillan, 1949[2]

	Blood glucose (mg/dl)	Serum cholesterol (mg/dl)	Percentage with atheroma
Control	121	959	88
Diabetic	278	1287	20
Alloxan recovered	120	469	100

McGill and Holman, 1949[3]

7.2). Another possible explanation was that the composition of the circulating lipids in the alloxan treated animals was abnormal[5]. It was suggested that alloxan diabetes results in a block 'in the conversion of the lipoproteins'. This must be an early reference to what is now known to be lipoprotein lipase deficiency in severe insulin-dependent diabetes. Treatment of alloxan diabetic rabbits or rats with insulin in doses sufficient to reduce glycosuria resulted in the same degree of atherosclerosis in the diabetics as in the non-diabetic controls[6,7] (Table 7.3).

Variable results have been obtained in other experiments[8–10]. In a study of different varieties of rats, some of which were prone to develop vascular lesions, alloxan diabetes had variable results depending on the breed of rat

Table 7.2 Effect of alloxan diabetes on experimental atherosclerosis in the cholesterol-fed rabbit[4]

	Blood glucose (mg/dl)	Serum cholesterol (mg/dl)	Atherosclerosis grade
Control	129	1728	2.9
Alloxan diabetic	545	2972	2.5
Pancreas protected	125	1378	3.4

Table 7.3 Effect of treatment of alloxan diabetic rabbits with insulin on experimental atherosclerosis[6]

	Serum cholesterol (mg/dl)	Atherosclerosis grade
Control	172	2.4
Untreated diabetic	205	1.3
Treated diabetic	185	2.2

and on the metabolic state of the animal. Thus, species differences in the response to severe insulin deficiency both with respect to lipid abnormalities and to vascular lesions probably exist. The effect of treatment of the experimental diabetes has not always been taken into account. Thus, a study entitled 'the effect of insulin deficiency' used alloxanized monkeys fed a high-fat diet but treated with up to 32 units of insulin per day. Insulin levels were not measured but it is unlikely that these animals were in fact insulin-deficient. They developed higher serum cholesterol or beta-lipoprotein levels and more vascular lesions than the controls[11].

The possibility that vascular lesions in rats with experimental diabetes might be related to the effect of diabetes on serum lipids has been considered[12-14]. Pancreatectomized rats had higher lipid levels and more vascular lesions than controls[12]. However, if the lipid levels in the pancreatectomized rats were adjusted by dietary means to similar levels to those in the control rats the vascular lesions in the diabetics and the controls were the same. This suggested that the increased vascular lesions in the diabetic animals were due to the high blood lipids. It also suggested that the diabetic artery is not more susceptible to ambient lipid concentrations than the non-diabetic artery. It was later found[15] that if the pancreatectomized rats were treated with insulin, serum cholesterol levels fell to levels which were similar to the levels of the animals which had been pancreatectomized but did not develop diabetes, but the vascular lesions were the same as those in the diabetic animals with the high blood lipid levels (Table 7.4). Thus, in the insulin-treated diabetic rat the normal relationship between serum cholesterol and vascular lesions was no longer present and the animals developed excess vascular lesions in relation to their serum cholesterol levels.

These experiments suggested the possibility that insulin might have a role in the development of the vascular lesions in diabetes. This was first studied indirectly in chickens[16]. In a large series of experiments on diet-induced vascular lesions in chickens it had been found that the vascular lesions regressed if the animals were restored to a normal diet, or could be prevented by oestrogen treatment of the animals. However, insulin, 10 units per day, inhibited the regression of atherosclerosis when the animals were returned to a normal diet and overcame the protective effect of

Table 7.4 Effect of pancreatectomy, diabetes and insulin on serum cholesterol and atherosclerosis in the rat. Treatment with insulin results in a dissociation between serum cholesterol and vascular lesions[15]

	Serum total cholesterol (mg/dl)	Cardiovascular score
Control	635 ± 87	1.5
Diabetic–saline	1863 ± 194	4.3
Diabetic–insulin	1014 ± 134	4.1
Pancreatectomized – non-diabetic	1178 ± 133	2.1

oestrogen. Insulin did not affect the induction of vascular lesions in animals fed a high-fat diet and the effects of insulin were not due to changes in the feeding patterns of the chickens. The effect of insulin on vascular lesions was also studied in alloxan diabetic dogs[17]. The right femoral artery was injected with crystalline insulin daily while the left was injected with saline. After 30 weeks the insulin-treated artery showed proliferative changes and a thickened media, and contained more cholesterol and fatty acid than the control artery. The muscle in the insulin-treated leg also contained more cholesterol than the control leg.

There has only been one study on the effect of insulin on the development of vascular lesions in non-diabetic animals fed a normal diet[18,19]. Free-living chickens were divided into two groups, one of which was injected four times per week with insulin zinc suspension while the other was injected with the same volume of a control solution for the insulin which contained all the constituents of the insulin solution except insulin. The animals fed *ad libitum* and after 19 weeks were sacrificed and the aortas examined. There was no difference in the weight change of the insulin-treated and control chickens and blood glucose levels were the same. Serum cholesterol and triglyceride were slightly higher in the insulin-treated birds. The aortas of the insulin-treated birds contained significantly more lipid-containing lesions than aortas of the control birds (Figure 7.1). There was no correlation between the extent of the vascular lesions and lipid and glucagon levels or insulin antibody titres. The spontaneous development of coronary artery lesions has also occurred in hyperinsulinaemic spiny mice fed on a normal diet[20]. In cholesterol-fed non-diabetic rabbits insulin increased aortic atherosclerosis, despite reducing serum lipid levels, and prevented regression of the vascular lesions when the animals were restored to a normal diet[21].

Overall, the results of studies of vascular lesions in animals with experimental diabetes suggest that insulin is necessary for the full development of experimental vascular lesions, that insulin deficiency may protect against vascular lesions, and that insulin may promote the development of the lesions.

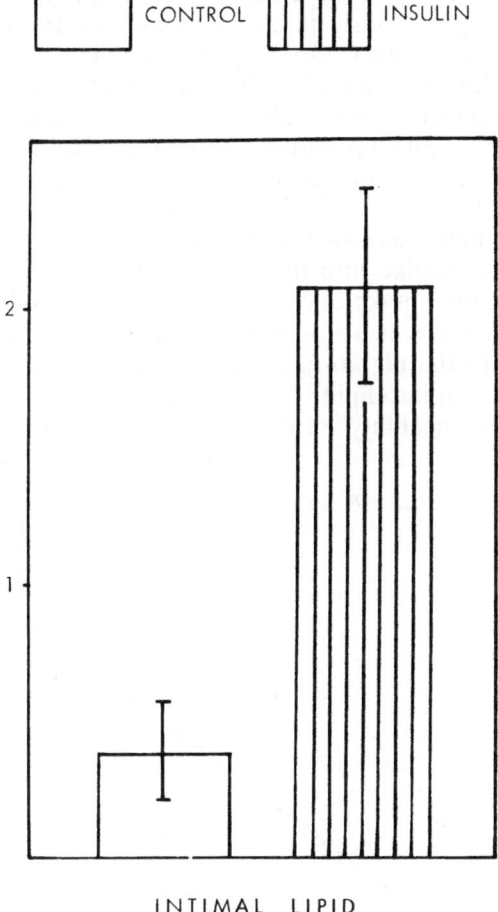

Figure 7.1   Intimal lipid in chickens injected with insulin and control chickens[18]

THE ARTERIAL WALL

The arterial wall is not merely an inert tube which transmits blood from one part of the body to another, but consists of metabolically active tissue which is of considerable total mass. The arterial wall has the capacity to synthesize all the constituents of the atheromatous plaque and metabolic activities such as oxygen and glucose metabolism can be measured.

Aortas removed from alloxan diabetic rats have decreased fatty acid and cholesterol synthesis and oxygen uptake[22,23]. On the other hand, provided all fatty adventitious tissue is removed, aortas incubated *in vitro* are resistant to the effects of insulin on lipid synthesis[24-27]. However, very large doses of insulin increased glycogen synthesis in bovine mesenteric artery[28] and glucose uptake in rat and rabbit aorta[29].

Despite the lack of an insulin effect on aortic lipid metabolism *in vitro*, insulin injected intravenously into rats stimulated the incorporation of glucose[30] and acetate[31] into aortic lipids. The lipids involved included triglyceride, cholesterol and phospholipid. Aortas removed from rats rendered insulin-deficient and diabetic with streptozotocin incorporated less labelled glucose into lipid than aortas of control non-diabetic rats[27]. The plasma insulin level in the rats and the glucose incorporation into lipids was positively correlated (Figure 7.2). Similarly, when insulin was injected into normal rats there was a significant correlation between plasma insulin levels and glucose uptake into the isolated aorta[32]. Insulin and diabetes have no effect on the uptake of cholesterol into the aorta[31,33,34].

A number of factors which modify the insulin sensitivity of the aorta have been described. In the pig aorta the sensitivity to insulin of glucose and acetate incorporation into lipid[35,36] was focal in nature and was only found in areas of low permeability[37,38]. Glucose utilization in isolated aortas of

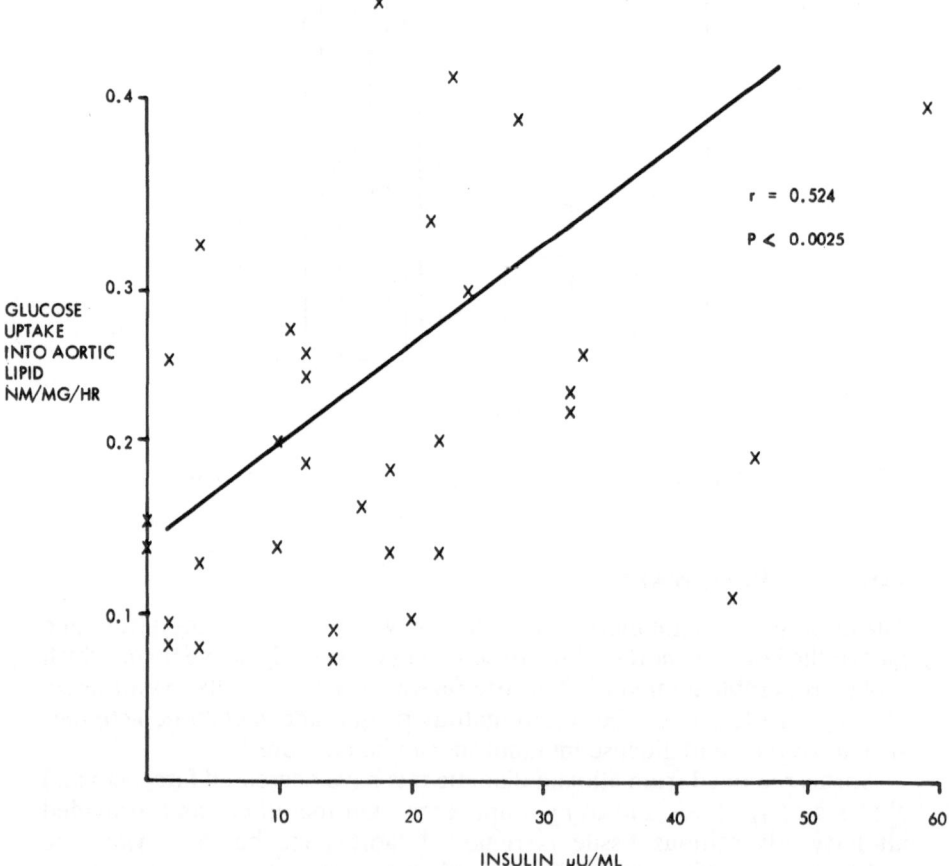

Figure 7.2 Relation of insulin levels to incorporation of glucose into aortic lipid in streptozotocin-treated rats[27]

spontaneous diabetic Chinese hamsters was decreased and restored to normal by high-dose insulin treatment[39]. Insulin sensitivity of the aorta is influenced by the nutritional status of the animal[40,41] and by treatment of spontaneous hypertension[42].

An explanation for the paradox that arterial tissue is insensitive to insulin when incubated *in vitro* but responds to changes in circulating insulin levels *in vivo* has recently been provided[43]. Using an ingenious perfusion system which allowed changes in intravascular pressure, it was shown that at low pressure insulin had no effect on the metabolism of the arterial media, but at high pressure insulin stimulated lipid synthesis from glucose in the media. This was the first demonstration of an interaction between haemodynamic forces and the response of the arterial wall to insulin.

Diabetes and insulin influence the activities of catabolic enzymes in the arterial wall. The aorta contains a hormone-sensitive lipase of similar activity to the hormone-sensitive lipase in adipose tissue. This is stimulated by catecholamines, inhibited by insulin, and increased in states of insulin deficiency according to some[44] but not all investigators[45,46]. Enzymes involved in carbohydrate metabolism are not uniformly affected by experimental diabetes and insulin[47]. Lysosomal hydrolase enzymes have been considered to play a role in atherosclerosis[48]. Deficiency of these enzymes will lead to impaired breakdown of intracellular substances including lipoproteins. Experimental diabetes, caused by either streptozotocin or alloxan, results in decreased hydrolase activity in the rat aorta[49]; activities were restored to normal by insulin.

CELL CULTURE STUDIES

The important arterial cells in the development of atherosclerosis are the endothelial cells of the intima and the smooth muscle cells of the media (Chapter 2). Methods are available for culturing both smooth muscle cells[50] and endothelial cells[51,52]. Studies of the effects of glucose, insulin and serum from diabetics on cultured endothelial and smooth muscle cells have been reported.

Insulin stimulates proliferation of smooth muscle cells grown from monkey[53], rat[54,55] and human[56] aortas (Figure 7.3) and DNA synthesis in smooth muscle cells from rat aortas[57]. The effects on cell proliferation were seen with concentrations of insulin as low as $10\,\mu U/ml$ while in the monkey smooth muscle cells removal of native insulin from the serum resulted in decreased proliferation compared to the same concentration of whole serum. Smooth muscle cells appear to be particularly sensitive to the proliferative effects of insulin. The cells lost their sensitivity to the proliferative effects of insulin when they had 'aged' *in vitro*[53,54]. Insulin also stimulates the incorporation of acetate into sterols in cultured rat smooth muscle cells[58] but physiological concentrations of glucagon had no effect on this process[59]. Insulin stimulates binding and degradation of LDL in cultured human fibroblasts but does not seem to have this effect on smooth muscle cells[60].

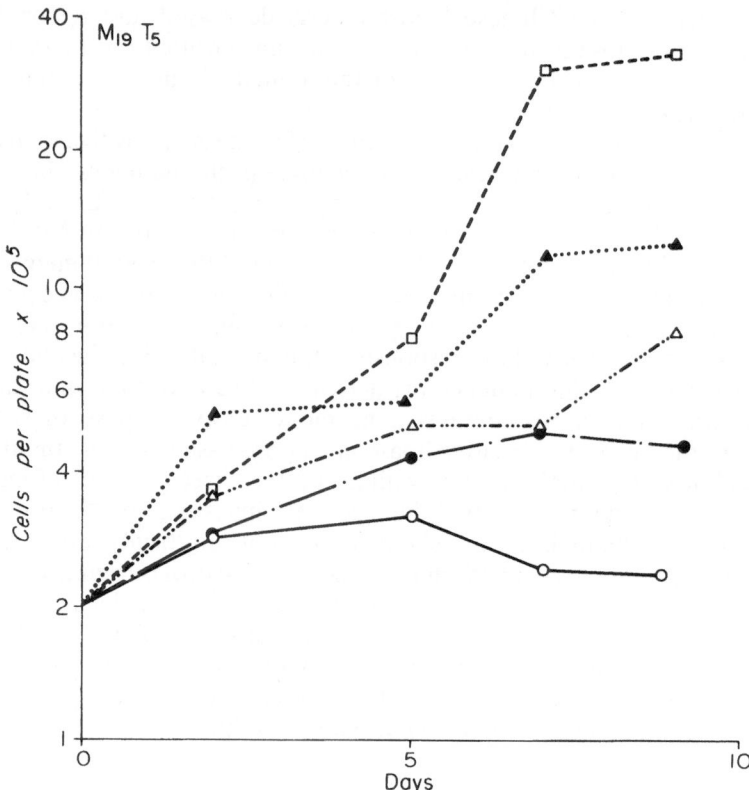

Figure 7.3 Effect of insulin on proliferation of cultured monkey aortic smooth muscle cells. All the cells were grown for 1 week in medium supplemented with 1% homologous monkey serum (not shown). They were then divided into five groups and grown in medium with 1% monkey serum (O), 1% serum with 100 (●), 1000 (△), or 10000 (▲) μU/ml insulin or 5% monkey serum (□)[53]

Human endothelial cells cultured from umbilical vein are resistant to the actions of insulin even in large concentrations[57] (Figure 7.4). Despite this, endothelial cell membranes contain insulin receptors[61,62]. The role of insulin receptors in the absence of insulin sensitivity is unknown.

Glucose has no effect on the proliferation of arterial smooth muscle cells[63]. This contrasts with its stimulating effect on fibroblast proliferation. On the other hand, glucose in concentrations found in diabetics inhibits the proliferation of cultured human endothelial cells[64] (Figure 7.5). This suggests that high ambient glucose concentrations might impair the healing response of endothelial cells to injury, and hence allow plasma constituents increased access to the inner layers of the artery.

The effect of diabetic serum on cultured cells has been studied by two methods. Rabbit aortic smooth muscle cells in primary culture grew better when exposed to serum from rabbits with experimental diabetes[65]. Serum from insulin-treated human diabetics had similar effects[66]. However, added

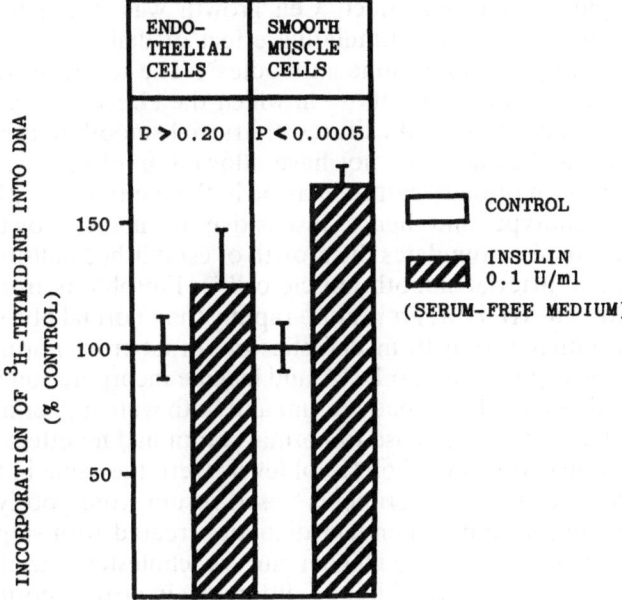

Figure 7.4   Effect of insulin on DNA synthesis in cultured human umbilical venous
endothelial cells and rat aortic smooth muscle cells [57]

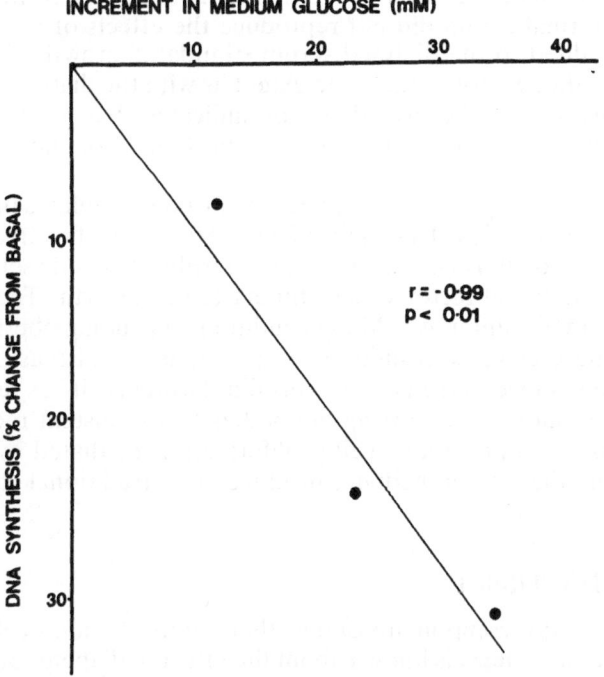

Figure 7.5   Effect of medium glucose concentration on DNA synthesis in cultured
human umbilical venous endothelial cells[64]

insulin or glucose had no effect. Cell growth was stimulated by added growth hormone[67] and the stimulating effect of diabetic serum could be blocked by anti-growth hormone antibodies[66]. The results of these studies are difficult to compare with those in which the effect of insulin has been demonstrated on established cultures of arterial smooth muscle cells. The experimental techniques may not have allowed an effect of insulin to be seen. Also cells in primary culture may be in the contractile rather than the synthetic phenotype and hence insensitive to many growth factors[68]. Diabetic serum also stimulates the growth of established cultures of human fibroblasts and arterial smooth muscle cells[69]. Fibroblasts from diabetics, both IDDM and NIDDM, grew more rapidly than normal fibroblasts when exposed to either serum from diabetics or serum from normal subjects. Thymidine incorporation into DNA and leucine incorporation into protein were both stimulated by diabetic serum and both were higher in fibroblasts from diabetics. Adding glucose to normal serum had no effect and growth hormone, triglyceride and cholesterol levels were the same in the diabetic and normal sera. Later experiments[70] used serum from poorly controlled non-ketotic, non-insulin-dependent diabetics treated with sulphonylureas or diet. The diabetic serum had higher glucose, cholesterol, triglyceride and insulin levels than the normal but no difference in growth hormone levels. Diabetic serum increased the growth of smooth muscle cells by 25–50%. Dialysis of the diabetic serum was performed, compounds of less than 12 000 daltons being removed. The dialysate had no effect by itself but was stimulatory when added to either normal or diabetic serum. Increasing the glucose in normal serum did not reproduce the effects of diabetic serum, but insulin added to the dialysed serum stimulated growth of the smooth muscle cells, though not to the same extent as with the diabetic serum. The molecular weight of the growth factor indicates that growth hormone, platelet-derived growth factors or lipoproteins are not the factors responsible.

The cell culture experiments suggest that insulin stimulates the growth of arterial smooth muscle cells and fibroblasts. However, the effect of normal serum on cell growth is not entirely due to insulin. Diabetic serum appears to have an additional factor which stimulates cell growth. The identity of this factor remains unknown. Many conditions, including obesity and mild diabetes, where elevated insulin levels are found are also associated with peripheral resistance to the action of insulin. However, it has recently been shown, using naturally occurring antibodies to the insulin receptor, that insulin's activity in promoting cell proliferation is mediated by a different receptor from that which mediates insulin's more traditional activities[71].

CONNECTIVE TISSUE

Of the three major components of the atheromatous lesion – cells, lipid and connective tissue – least is known about the effect of diabetes on connective tissue metabolism. Connective tissue has a number of functions which might be important in the pathogenesis of atherosclerosis[72]. These include

(1) the maintenance of the structural integrity of the artery;
(2) the maintenance of viscoelastic properties of the arterial wall;
(3) the regulation of permeability of the arterial wall;
(4) lipid entrapment and clearance;
(5) haemostatic mechanisms.

Proteoglycans can be synthesized and secreted by arterial smooth muscle cells[72-74]. There have been few reported studies of the effect of diabetes or insulin on this process. A practical difficulty in interpreting the results of such studies is that insulin stimulates proliferation of arterial smooth muscle cells[53] and the effects of cell proliferation[72] cannot easily be distinguished from the effects of the hormone. However, insulin in physiological concentrations stimulates proteoglycan synthesis in cultured chondrocytes in the absence of a significant effect on DNA synthesis[75]. On the other hand, insulin had no effect on proteoglycan synthesis in cultured human aortic smooth muscle cells[76]. In dogs made diabetic with alloxan glycosaminoglycan (GAG) content of large and medium-sized arteries was altered but not in a uniform fashion with respect to either GAG or specific arteries[77]. Diabetic dogs treated with insulin showed an increase in certain GAGs in some arteries, particularly the coronary arteries[78]. The effect of insulin was confirmed in hypophysectomized dogs which had hyperinsulinaemia without hyperglycaemia[78].

Collagen[79-82] and elastin[79,83,84] are synthesized by arterial smooth muscle cells. Diabetic serum stimulates the formation of procollagen I but not procollagen III in cultured rabbit aortic smooth muscle cells[85]. Fibronectin formation is also stimulated by diabetic serum. Glucose and insulin had no effect on procollagen I biosynthesis but the process was stimulated by growth hormone. Fibroblasts grown from diabetics synthesize more collagen than normal fibroblasts[86].

The evidence, though sparse, is consistent with diabetes having an effect on connective tissue metabolism in the arterial wall. In particular, insulin may stimulate the formation of proteoglycans in a way which contributes to the pathogenesis of atherosclerosis.

PROSTACYCLIN

The role of prostacyclin (PGI_2), a prostaglandin derived from arachidonic acid, has been discussed in Chapter 4. Prostacyclin is made and secreted by endothelial cells and is a potent inhibitor of platelet aggregation. Prostacyclin was first described in 1976[87] and there have only been a few studies of the effects of experimental diabetes on its activity. Streptozotocin diabetes in rats[88,89] and swine[90] results in a decrease in aortic prostacyclin production. Thromboxane B_2 production was increased in streptozotocin diabetic rats[88]. Prostacyclin synthesis returned to normal when the experimental diabetes was treated with insulin[89] or by islet tissue transplantation[88]. The latter procedure also restored thromboxane synthesis to normal.

The findings in experimental diabetes are consistent with those in human diabetes discussed in Chapter 4. The role of prostacyclin and thromboxane in atherogenesis is not clear. However, if an early stage in the development of atherosclerosis is platelet aggregation on an injured endothelium, with release of the platelet-derived growth factor[91], then factors which influence platelet aggregation may affect this process. The changes in prostacyclin and thromboxane synthesis in both human and experimental diabetes would tend to encourage platelet aggregation.

CONCLUSIONS

Diabetes has widespread effects on carbohydrate, lipid and protein metabolism and is associated with abnormal insulin secretion and activity, with changes in counter-regulatory hormones and with abnormalities in cell function which may be genetic in origin. It is naive to expect that any one abnormality is responsible for the association of diabetes with atherosclerosis, also a highly complex disorder. Most of the experimental techniques described in this chapter only reproduce some of the features of human diabetes. Thus while knowledge of the biology of the arterial wall has been gained, it is difficult to fit this into the total picture of human diabetes.

With respect to experimental diabetes and the arterial wall, some conclusions can be drawn.

(1) Hyperglycaemia does not result in arterial lesions in the absence of circulating insulin, despite hyperlipidaemia.
(2) Administration of insulin promotes the development of arterial lesions in animals fed a normal diet and inhibits regression of lesions in cholesterol-fed animals.
(3) Insulin promotes lipid synthesis in the arterial wall. This process may not be uniform throughout the arterial tree and may be modified by intra-arterial pressure.
(4) Insulin stimulates proliferation of smooth muscle cells but has no effect on endothelial cells.
(5) Glucose inhibits proliferation of endothelial cells but has no effect on smooth muscle cells.
(6) Diabetic serum contains a factor which stimulates smooth muscle cell proliferation. This substance may not be glucose or insulin.
(7) Insulin may stimulate proteoglycan synthesis.
(8) Diabetes is associated with decreased prostacyclin and increased thromboxane activity.

Using this information, a hypothesis linking diabetes and atherosclerosis can be proposed[64]. Hyperglycaemia inhibits endothelial cell replication, potentiating or even causing endothelial injury. This allows platelet aggregation on subendothelial tissue and exposure of smooth muscle cells to plasma. Growth factors from platelets and plasma, including insulin, stimulate smooth muscle cell proliferation and connective tissue synthesis. Lipoproteins are taken up by the smooth muscle cells and infiltrate the extracellular tissues.

This scheme takes account of the experimental evidence reviewed in this chapter and is also consistent with the clinical and epidemiological features of diabetes and atherosclerosis. In particular, it explains the threshold relationship between blood glucose levels and atherosclerosis, and the fact that risk factors have the same relationship to atherosclerosis in diabetics and non-diabetics.

References

1. Dragstedt, L. R., Clark, D. E., Julian, O. C., Vermeulen, C. and Goodpasture, W. C. (1940). Arteriosclerosis in pancreatic diabetes. *Surgery*, **8**, 353
2. Duff, G. L. and McMillan, G. C. (1949). The effect of alloxan diabetes on experimental atherosclerosis in the rabbit. I. The inhibition of experimental atherosclerosis in alloxan diabetes. II. The effect of alloxan diabetes on the retrogression of experimental cholesterol atherosclerosis. *J. Exp. Med.*, **89**, 611
3. McGill, H. C. and Holman, R. L. (1949). The influence of alloxan diabetes on cholesterol atheromatosis in the rabbit. *Proc. Soc. Exp. Biol. Med.*, **72**, 72
4. Cook, D. L., Mills, L. M. and Green, O. M. (1954). The mechanism of alloxan protection in experimental atherosclerosis. *J. Exp. Med.*, **99**, 119
5. Pierce, F. T. (1952). The relationship of serum lipoproteins to atherosclerosis in the cholesterol fed alloxanised rabbit. *Circulation*, **5**, 401
6. Duff, G. L., Brechin, D. J. H. and Findelstein, W. E. (1954). The effect of alloxan diabetes on experimental cholesterol atherosclerosis in the rabbit. IV. The effect of insulin therapy on the inhibition of atherosclerosis in the alloxan-diabetic rabbit. *J. Exp. Med.*, **100**, 371
7. Beveridge, J. M. R. and Johnson, S. E. (1950). Studies on diabetic rats: production of cardiovascular and renal disease in diabetic rats. *Br. J. Exp. Pathol.*, **31**, 285
8. Kalant, N. and Harland, W. A. (1961). The effect of an atherogenic diet on normal and alloxan diabetic rats. *Can. Med. Assoc. J.*, **84**, 251
9. Kalant, N., Teitelbaum, J. I., Cooperberg, A. A. and Harland, W. A. (1964). Dietary atherogenesis in alloxan diabetes. *J. Lab. Clin. Med.*, **63**, 147
10. Still, W. J. S., Martin, J. M. and Gregor, W. H. (1964). The effect of alloxan diabetes on experimental atherosclerosis in the rat. *Exp. Mol. Pathol.*, **3**, 141
11. Lehner, N. D. M., Clarkson, T. E. and Lofland, H. B. (1971). The effect of insulin deficiency, hypothyroidism, and hypertension on atherosclerosis in the squirrel monkey. *Exp. Mol. Pathol.*, **15**, 230
12. Wilson, R. B., Martin, J. M. and Hartroft, W. S. (1967). Evaluation of the relative pathogenic roles of diabetes and serum cholesterol levels in the development of cardiovascular lesions in rats. *Diabetes*, **16**, 71
13. Reinila, A., Akerblom, H. K. and Scow, R. O. (1980). Accumulation of lipid in muscular arteries of short-term diabetic rats. *Diabetologia*, **19**, 529
14. Wexler, B. C. and Sangrey, D. G. (1980). Good versus moderate regulation of alloxan-induced diabetes in arteriosclerotic and nonarteriosclerotic rats. *Diabetologia*, **19**, 242
15. Wilson, R. B., Martin, J. M. and Hartroft, W. S. (1969). Failure of insulin therapy to prevent cardiovascular lesions in diabetic rats fed an atherogenic diet. *Diabetes*, **18**, 225
16. Stamler, J., Pick, R. and Katz, L. N. (1960). Effect of insulin in the induction and regression of atherosclerosis in the chick. *Circ. Res.*, **8**, 572
17. Cruz, A. B., Amatuzio, D. S., Grande, F. and Hay, L. J. (1961). Effect of intra-arterial insulin on tissue cholesterol and fatty acids in alloxan-diabetic dogs. *Circ. Res.*, **9**, 39
18. Stout, R. W. (1970). Development of vascular lesions in insulin-treated animals fed a normal diet. *Br. Med. J.*, **3**, 685
19. Stout, R. W., Buchanan, K. D. and Vallance-Owen, J. (1973). The relationship of arterial disease and glucagon metabolism in insulin-treated chickens. *Atherosclerosis*, **18**, 153
20. Renold, A. E., Gonet, A. E., Stauffacher, W. and Jeanrenaud, B. (1968). Laboratory animals with spontaneous diabetes and/or obesity: suggested suitability for the study of spontaneous atherosclerosis. *Prog. Biochem. Pharmacol.*, **4**, 363

21. Marquie, G. (1978). Effect of insulin in the induction and regression of experimental cholesterol atherosclerosis in the rabbit. *Postgrad. Med. J.*, **54**, 80

22. Foster, D. W. and Siperstein, M. D. (1960). Effect of diabetes on cholesterol and fatty acid synthesis in the rat aorta. *Am. J. Physiol.*, **198**, 25

23. Wong, R. K. L. and Van Bruggen, J. T. (1962). Lipid metabolism in the diabetic rat. VI. Metabolic activity of the aorta. *Acta Physiol. Latin Am.*, **12**, 390

24. Wertheimer, H. E. and Ben-Tor, V. (1962). Influence of diabetes on carbohydrate metabolism of aortic tissue. *Diabetes*, **11**, 422

25. Mulcahy, P. D. and Winegrad, A. I. (1962). Effects of insulin and alloxan diabetes on glucose metabolism in rabbit aortic tissue. *Am. J. Physiol.*, **203**, 1038

26. Urrutia, G., Beaven, D. W. and Cahill, G. F. (1962). Metabolism of glucose-U-C14 in rat aorta *in vitro*. *Metabolism*, **11**, 530

27. Stout, R. W., Buchanan, K. D. and Vallance-Owen, J. (1972). Arterial lipid metabolism in relation to blood glucose and plasma insulin in rats with streptozotocin-induced diabetes. *Diabetologia*, **8**, 398

28. Lundholm, L. and Mohme-Lundholm, E. (1962). Effect of insulin on the carbohydrate metabolism of smooth muscle. *Acta Physiol. Scand.*, **57**, 130

29. Arnqvist, H. J. (1971). Studies of monosaccharide permeability of arterial tissue and intestinal smooth muscle; effects of insulin. *Acta Physiol. Scand.*, **83**, 247

30. Stout, R. W. (1968). Insulin stimulated lipogenesis in arterial tissue in relation to diabetes and atheroma. *Lancet*, **2**, 702

31. Stout, R. W. (1969). Insulin stimulation of cholesterol synthesis by arterial tissue. *Lancet*, **2**, 467

32. Capron, L., Housset, E. and Hartmann, L. (1980). Effects of *in vitro* and *in vivo* exposure to insulin upon glucose carbon accumulation in rat aorta: different patterns of response for intima–media and adventitia. *Metabolism*, **29**, 859

33. Hruza, Z. (1971). Effect of endocrine factors on cholesterol turnover in young and old rats. *Exp. Gerontol.*, **6**, 199

34. Matsuda, I. and Kalant, M. (1966). Effect of alloxan diabetes on cholesterol flux into aorta. *Diabetes*, **15**, 604

35. Somer, J. B. and Schwartz, C. J. (1976). Regulation of lipid metabolism in the normal pig aorta. 2. Influence of insulin and epinephrine on lipid synthesis from (1–^{14}C) acetate. *Atherosclerosis*, **23**, 215

36. Somer, J. B. and Schwartz, C. J. (1976). Focal differences in lipid metabolism of the young pig aorta. IV. Influence of insulin and epinephrine on lipogenesis from (^{14}C)-U-glucose. *Exp. Mol. Pathol.*, **24**, 129

37. Somer, J. B. and Schwartz, C. J. (1976). Regulation of lipid metabolism in the normal pig aorta. *Atherosclerosis*, **23**, 201, 215

38. Somer, J. B., Gerrity, R. G. and Schwartz, C. J. (1976). Focal differences in lipid metabolism of the young pig aorta. III. Influence of insulin on lipogenesis from (1–^{14}C) acetate. *Exp. Mol. Pathol.*, **24**, 1

39. Chobanian, A. V., Gerritsen, G. C., Brecher, P. I. and McCombs, L. (1974). Aortic glucose metabolism in the diabetic Chinese hamster. *Diabetologia*, **10**, 589

40. O'Dea, K., Klapovitz, H. and Marino, A. (1977). Effect of meal feeding on insulin sensitivity and incorporation of (U^{14}C) glucose into lipids in rat aorta. *J. Nutr.*, **107**, 1896

41. O'Dea, K. (1978). Effects of fasting and refeeding on the in vitro insulin sensitivity of rat aorta. *Horm. Metab. Res.*, **10**, 52

42. O'Dea, K., Tank, C., Klapovitz, H. and Marino, A. J. (1978). Development of insulin sensitivity in rat aorta after chronic propranolol treatment. *Eur. J. Pharmacol.*, **47**, 63

43. Capron, L., Philippe, M., Guilmot, J.-L., Fiessinger, J.-N. and Housset, E. (1981). Effects of insulin exposure upon the metabolism of rat aortic media: influence of hydrostatic forces. *Arteriosclerosis*, **1**, 345

44. Mahler, R. (1971). The effect of diabetes and insulin on biochemical reactions of the arterial wall. *Acta Diabet. Lat.*, **8**, 63

45. Chmelar, M. and Chmelarova, M. (1969). Lipolytic effect of insulin and other hormones in vitro in aortic tissue of experimental animals. *Experientia*, **24**, 1118

46. Orimo, H., Sakurada, T., Ito, H., Okabe, H., Noma, A. and Murakami, M. (1975). Lipid metabolism in aorta of rats with streptozotocin-induced diabetes. *Artery*, **1**, 335

47. Agren, A. and Arnqvist, H. J. (1981). Influence of diabetes on enzyme activities in rat aorta. *Diabete Metab. (Paris)*, **7**, 19
48. Wolinsky, H. and Fowler, S. (1978). Participation of lysosomes in atherosclerosis. *N. Engl. J. Med.*, **299**, 1173
49. Wolinsky, H., Goldfischer, S., Capron, L., Capron, F., Coltoff-Schiller, B. and Kasak, L. (1978). Hydrolase activities in the rat aorta. 1. Effects of diabetes mellitus and insulin treatment. *Circ. Res.*, **47**, 821
50. Ross, R. (1971). The smooth muscle cell. II. Growth of smooth muscle in culture and formation of elastic fibres. *J. Cell Biol.*, **50**, 172
51. Jaffe, E. A., Nachman, R. L., Becker, C. G. and Minick, C. R. (1973). Culture of human endothelial cells derived from umbilical veins. Identification by morphologic and immunologic criteria. *J. Clin. Invest.*, **52**, 2745
52. Gimbrone, M. A. Jr., Cotran, R. S. and Folkman, J. (1974). Human vascular endothelial cells in culture. *J. Cell Biol.*, **60**, 673
53. Stout, R. W., Bierman, E. L. and Ross, R. (1975). Effect of insulin on the proliferation of cultured primate arterial smooth muscle cells. *Circ. Res.*, **36**, 319
54. Pfeifle, B., Ditschuneit, H. H. and Ditschuneit, H. (1980). Insulin as a cellular growth regulator of rat arterial smooth muscle cells *in vitro*. *Horm. Metab. Res.*, **12**, 381
55. Weinstein, R., Stemerman, M. B. and Maciag, T. (1981). Hormonal requirements for growth of arterial smooth muscle cells in vitro: an endocrine approach to atherosclerosis. *Science*, **212**, 818
56. Pfeifle, B. and Ditschuneit, H. (1981). Effect of insulin on growth of cultured human arterial smooth muscle cells. *Diabetologia*, **20**, 155
57. Taggart, H. and Stout, R. W. (1980). Control of DNA synthesis in cultured vascular endothelial and smooth muscle cells. *Atherosclerosis*, **37**, 549
58. Stout, R. W. (1977). The effect of insulin and glucose on sterol synthesis in cultured rat arterial smooth muscle cells. *Atherosclerosis*, **27**, 271
59. Stout, R. W. (1978). Relative insensitivity to glucagon of sterol synthesis in cultured rat aortic smooth muscle cells. Effect of dibutyryl cyclic AMP. *Diabetologia*, **15**, 323
60. Chait, A., Bierman, E. L. and Albers, J. J. (1978). Regulatory role of insulin in the degradation of low density lipoprotein by cultured human skin fibroblasts. *Biochim. Biophys. Acta*, **529**, 292
61. Bar, R. S., Hoak, J. C. and Peacock, M. L. (1978). Insulin receptors in human endothelial cells: identification and characterisation. *J. Clin. Endocrinol. Metab.*, **47**, 699
62. Bar, R. S., Peacock, M. L., Spanheimer, R. G., Veenstra, R. and Hoak, J. C. (1980). Differential binding of insulin to human arterial and venous endothelial cells in primary culture. *Diabetes*, **29**, 991
63. Turner, J. L. and Bierman, E. L. (1978). Effects of glucose and sorbitol on proliferation of cultured human skin fibroblasts and arterial smooth muscle cells. *Diabetes*, **27**, 583
64. Stout, R. W. (1982). Glucose inhibits replication of cultured human endothelial cells. *Diabetologia*. (In press)
65. Ledet, T., Fischer-Dzoga, K. and Wissler, R. W. (1976). Growth of rabbit aortic smooth muscle cells cultured in media containing diabetic and hyperlipemic serum. *Diabetes*, **25**, 207
66. Ledet, T. (1976). Growth hormone stimulates the growth of arterial medial cells in vitro. *Diabetes*, **25**, 1011
67. Ledet, T. (1977). Growth hormone antiserum suppresses the growth effect of diabetic serum. *Diabetes*, **26**, 798
68. Chamley-Campbell, J. H. and Campbell, G. R. (1981). What controls smooth muscle phenotype? *Atherosclerosis*, **40**, 347
69. Koschinsky, T., Bunting, C. E., Schwippert, B. and Gries, F. A. (1979). Increased growth of human fibroblasts and arterial smooth muscle cells from diabetic patients related to diabetic serum factors and cell origin. *Atherosclerosis*, **33**, 245
70. Koschinsky, T., Bunting, C. E., Schwippert, B. and Gries, F. A. (1980). Increased growth stimulation of fibroblasts from diabetics by diabetic serum factors of low molecular weight. *Atherosclerosis*, **37**, 311
71. King, G. L., Kahn, C. R., Rechler, M. M. and Nissley, S. P. (1980). Direct demonstration of separate receptors for growth and metabolic activities of insulin and multiplication-

stimulating activity (an insulin-like growth factor) using antibodies to the insulin receptor. *J. Clin. Invest.*, **66**, 130

72. Wight, T. N. (1980). Vessel proteoglycans and thrombogenesis. In Spaet, T. H. (ed.) *Progress in Hemostasis and Thrombosis*. Vol. 5. (New York: Grune & Stratton)

73. Wight, T. N. and Ross, R. (1975). Proteoglycans in primate arteries. II. Synthesis and secretion of glycosaminoglycans by arterial smooth muscle cells in culture. *J. Cell Biol.*, **67**, 675

74. Deudon, E., Breton, M., Berrou, E. and Picard, J. (1980). Metabolism of glycosaminoglycans in cultured smooth muscle cells from pig aorta. *Biochemie*, **62**, 811

75. Stevens, R. L., Nissley, S. P., Kimura, J. H., Rechler, M. M., Caplan, A. I. and Hascall, V. C. (1981). Effects of insulin and multiplication-stimulating activity on proteoglycan biosynthesis in chondrocytes from the swarm rat chondrosarcoma. *J. Biol. Chem.*, **256**, 2045

76. Ronnemaa, T., Jarvelainen, H., Lehtonen, A. *et al.* (1980). Serum lipoprotein composition, hormones and the synthesis of glycosaminoglycans by human aortic smooth muscle cells. *Artery*, **8**, 323

77. Sirek, O. V., Sirek, A. and Cukerman, E. (1980). Arterial glycosaminoglycans in diabetic dogs. *Blood Vessels*, **17**, 271

78. Sirek, O. V., Sirek, A. and Cukerman, E. (1981). Intermittent hyperinsulinaemia and arterial glycosaminoglycans in dogs. *Diabetologia*, **21**, 154

79. Ross, R. and Klebanoff, S. J. (1971). The smooth muscle cell. I. *In vivo* synthesis of connective tissue proteins. *J. Cell Biol.*, **50**, 159

80. Burke, J. M. and Ross, R. (1977). Collagen synthesis by monkey arterial smooth muscle cells during proliferation and quiescence in culture. *Exp. Cell Res.*, **107**, 387

81. Layman, D. L., Epstein, E. H., Dodson, R. F. and Titus, J. L. (1977). Biosynthesis of type I and III collagens by cultured smooth muscle cells from human aorta. *Proc. Natl. Acad. Sci. USA*, **74**, 671

82. Salcedo, L. L. and Franzblau, C. (1981). Collagen synthesis and accumulation in long-term rabbit aortic smooth muscle cell cultures. *In Vitro*, **17**, 114

83. Abraham, P. A., Smith, D. W. and Carnes, W. H. (1974). Synthesis of soluble elastin by aortic medial cells in culture. *Biochem. Biophys. Res. Commun.*, **58**, 597

84. Narayanan, A. S., Sandberg, L. B., Ross, R. and Layman, D. L. (1976). The smooth muscle cell. III. Elastin synthesis in arterial smooth muscle cell culture. *J. Cell Biol.*, **68**, 411

85. Ledet, T. and Luust, J. (1980). Arterial procollagen type I, type III and fibronectin. Effects of diabetic serum, glucose, insulin, ketones and growth hormone studied on rabbit aortic myomedial cell cultures. *Diabetes*, **29**, 964

86. Smith, B. D. and Silbert, C. K. (1981). Fibronectin and collagen of cultured skin fibroblasts in diabetes mellitus. *Biochem. Biophys. Res. Commun.*, **100**, 275

87. Moncada, S., Gryglewski, R., Bunting, S. and Vane, J. R. (1976). An enzyme isolated from arteries transforms prostaglandin endoperoxides to an unstable substance that inhibits platelet aggregation. *Nature (London)*, **263**, 663

88. Gerrard, J. M., Stuart, M. J., Rao, G. H. R. *et al.* (1980). Alteration in the balance of prostaglandin and thromboxane synthesis in diabetic rats. *J. Lab. Clin. Invest.*, **95**, 950

89. Harrison, H. E., Reece, A. H. and Johnson, M. (1980). Effect of insulin treatment on prostacyclin in experimental diabetes. *Diabetologia*, **18**, 65

90. Silberbauer, K., Clopath, P., Sinzinger, H. and Schernthaner, G. (1980). Effect of experimentally induced diabetes on swine vascular prostacyclin (PGI_2) synthesis. *Artery*, **8**, 30

91. Ross, R. (1981). Atherosclerosis: a problem of the biology of arterial wall cells and their interactions with blood components. *Arteriosclerosis*, **1**, 293

8
Diabetes and atherosclerosis – conclusions

Diabetes mellitus is associated with accelerated atherosclerosis. The association occurs in the absence of treatment of diabetes and is not influenced by treatment. The presence of diabetes removes the normal female protection against atherosclerosis. Risk factors have the same relationship to atherosclerosis in diabetics as in non-diabetics, but the increased incidence of atherosclerosis in diabetes is not entirely explained by an increased prevalence of risk factors. In non-diabetics, high plasma insulin levels are associated with an increased incidence of cardiovascular disease and insulin has actions on the arterial wall which may promote atherogenesis.

Despite the large amount of information on diabetes and atherosclerosis that has become available, a number of important questions remain unanswered.

(1) Is atherosclerosis a complication of diabetes or an associated condition? The evidence available does not allow a definite answer to this question. On the one hand, hyperglycaemia in the absence of diabetes is associated with accelerated atherosclerosis and high ambient glucose levels inhibit endothelial cell replication. On the other hand, reduction of blood sugar levels does not prevent the development of cardiovascular disease. The results of genetic studies are consistent with the link between diabetes and atherosclerosis being other than cause and effect, but further information is required. Studies of the function of arterial endothelial and smooth muscle cells from diabetics are also needed. It is of course possible that hyperglycaemia and atherosclerosis are related in two ways – as cause and effect and as genetically related conditions.

(2) What is the relation of risk factors to atherosclerosis in diabetes? Epidemiological studies have shown that the relation of risk factors to atherosclerosis is the same in diabetics as in non-diabetics. However, diabetics who develop cardiovascular disease have rarely been compared with age- and sex-matched diabetics without macro-

93

angiopathy. Thus, while it seems that the presence of risk factors does not entirely account for the increased prevalence of atherosclerosis in diabetics, there is little information on the importance of risk factors in the diabetic.

(3) What is the role of insulin in atherosclerosis in diabetics? The prospective studies that have revealed high insulin levels as a risk factor for atherosclerosis have been carried out in non-diabetics. There is no information on the predictive effect of high insulin levels in diabetics. The clinical, epidemiological and experimental evidence is strong enough to make studies of this question urgent.

(4) Have abnormalities of other hormones a role in atherosclerosis in diabetics? There is minimal and largely negative information on glucagon, but no information on the relationship of the newly described gastro-entero-pancreatic hormones in diabetes and atherosclerosis.

(5) What is the role of abnormalities in coagulation and in arachidonic acid metabolites in vascular disease in diabetes? The available evidence suggests that platelet function is abnormal in diabetics. With respect to atherosclerosis, studies of the effect of diabetes on the platelet-derived growth factor are important. The isolation of this growth factor and the development of assays should make these studies possible.

SEX HORMONES

SEX HORMONES

9
Atherosclerosis in males and females

THE SEX INCIDENCE OF ATHEROSCLEROSIS

Ischaemic heart disease is commoner in young men than in young women[1].
In England and Wales in 1973 there were 1942 deaths from coronary heart
disease in women aged 30–34 compared to 10 692 in men during the same
period[2]. However, after the age of about 50 years the incidence of
ischaemic heart disease in men and women tends to equalize and after
about 70 the incidences are much the same.

Most of the information on the sex incidence of ischaemic heart disease is
based on mortality rates reported in the Registrar General's annual returns
or similar statistics from other parts of the world. Such statistics are
notoriously unreliable. They are usually based on a clinical diagnosis of the
cause of death and if the death has been sudden, adequate documentation
of the presence of ischaemic heart disease may not have been possible.
Furthermore, even if fatal ischaemic heart disease is more common in men
than in women this does not necessarily mean that the difference is due to
atherosclerosis. Other factors, including thrombosis and the ability of the
heart to withstand an episode of coronary occlusion, may contribute to the
difference.

In the Framingham study women developed considerably less coronary
heart disease than men (Table 9.1). Indeed women developed coronary
heart disease at the rates of men about 10 years their juniors[3,4]. However,
the frequency of risk factors for atherosclerosis was similar in the two sexes
and the relationship of risk factors to coronary artery disease and cerebral
vascular disease was the same in males and females[5]. Vascular disease of
the brain occurred at similar rates in men and women at all ages[5]. This is
due to a much smaller rate of cerebral vascular disease in men compared
with myocardial infarction (Table 9.2). Thus, the rates of cerebral vascular
disease in men and in women and myocardial infarction in women are all
approximately the same.

In a Scandinavian study[6] it was found that the prevalence of myocardial
infarction was higher in men than in women although the frequency of

Table 9.1 Incidence of cardiovascular disease by age and sex (the Framingham study 20 year follow-up[4])

| Age | Rate per 1000 per year | | Ratio |
| | Men | Women | |
(years)			M : F
29–34	3.4	0.8	4.5 : 1
35–39	2.9	0.7	4.1 : 1
40–44	5.7	1.3	4.4 : 1
45–49	9.1	3.1	2.9 : 1
50–54	16.5	6.1	2.7 : 1
55–59	25.1	10.2	2.5 : 1
60–64	27.6	18.1	1.5 : 1
65–69	26.7	22.1	1.2 : 1
70–74	37.8	26.2	1.4 : 1
75–79	53.0	50.4	1.1 : 1

Table 9.2 Incidence per 1000 of cerebrovascular disease and myocardial infarction by age and sex (the Framingham study, 12-year follow-up[5])

Age at entry	Cerebrovascular disease	Myocardial infarction
Men		
30–39	2.4	27.9
40–49	11.7	57.1
50–59	24.6	98.9
Women		
30–39	1.0	1.9
40–49	7.4	7.3
50–59	26.7	25.3

angina pectoris was the same. This paradoxical finding has a number of possible explanations. It may indicate that the factors causing occlusion of the vessel may differ in males and females but the underlying vascular disease is the same, or it may be that women are more likely to develop chest pain with ischaemic heart disease. The incidence of myocardial infarction was 8 times higher in men than women in this population.

The question of whether the difference in ischaemic heart disease incidence in men and women in the younger age groups is due to atherosclerosis is difficult to answer clinically. The fact that cerebral vascular disease had the same incidence in males and females at all ages is against atherosclerosis being the cause, although it is possible that atherosclerosis affects different vessels in different ways and develops at different rates in different parts of the body. Studies of changes in mortality patterns have suggested that there are important differences in the pathogenesis of stroke and ischaemic heart disease and that they should not be regarded as manifestations of the same disease[7]. There are also differences in associated biochemical abnormalities in that plasma oestrogen levels are raised in men with myocardial infarction[8,9] but are unchanged in stroke[10]. Stroke is also more closely associated with raised blood pressure and less closely associated with abnormal serum lipids[5].

AUTOPSY STUDIES

Autopsy studies provide some information on the sex difference in the incidence of atherosclerosis. However modern quantitative techniques have rarely been employed in these studies. For example, more myocardial infarctions were found at post mortem in men than in women under the age of 50 and no difference over the age of 50, but there was no mention as to whether this was due to a difference in the extent of atherosclerosis[11]. In the Oxford study[12] it was found that women of a given age had arterial lesions of aorta and coronary arteries of a severity similar to that found in men a decade younger. On the other hand, females with cardiac infarction showed a pattern of atherosclerosis which was comparable with that of unselected females 10 years older than themselves. Stenosis of the coronary arteries was more common in men than women at all ages up to the age of 75. The Oxford study therefore provided evidence that atherosclerosis develops more slowly in women than in men at least up to the age of 75. In a study of sudden and unexpected deaths due to atherosclerotic heart disease, there were less coronary heart disease deaths in females but the proportion of deaths which were sudden was the same in males and females[13]. This suggests that epidemiological and clinical studies of cardiac death may reflect the incidence of atherosclerosis. A Scandinavian autopsy study of 1567 subjects aged 10 and over who died during an 18-month period showed that males had more atherosclerosis of the aorta up to the age of 70 and more complicated lesions at all ages[14]. Differences were even more marked in the coronary arteries where males had more atherosclerosis up to the age of 80 and also more complicated lesions. Females lagged by 10–15 years in the frequency of atherosclerosis in the coronary arteries. Males also had more peripheral artery atherosclerosis but there was little difference between the sexes in the extent of cerebral atherosclerosis.

   The largest autopsy study of atherosclerosis has been the International Atherosclerosis Project[15]. In this study the relationship of female sex to atherosclerosis depended on race, the arteries studied, the age of the subject, the type of lesion and the average severity of the lesions. Overall there was no sex difference in the frequency or extent of raised aortic lesions. However, in regions of the world where the overall prevalence of atherosclerosis is high males had more coronary atherosclerosis than females. There was also slightly more cerebral atherosclerosis in men than in women. On the other hand, more fatty streaks were found in the coronary arteries and aortae of young women than young men. In areas of the world where the overall prevalence of atherosclerosis is low, a difference between males and females was not found. This study suggests that where the prevalence of atherosclerosis is high then either the female sex has protective effect or the male an accelerating effect.

A weakness in all studies of atherosclerosis in younger people is that the number of subjects, particularly young women, has been small and hence firm conclusions are difficult to make. However, the autopsy studies are consistent in showing more atherosclerosis of the coronary arteries and aortae of young men than young women in areas where the incidence of atherosclerosis is high. The fact that where atherosclerosis is less common, the sex incidence is equal, suggests that a high incidence of atherosclerosis is related to a factor that selectively influences men. The reason why the cerebral arteries do not share in the differential sex incidence of atherosclerosis is unknown.

CHARACTERISTICS OF YOUNGER WOMEN WHO DEVELOP CORONARY ARTERY DISEASE

Ischaemic heart disease is rare in young women. However, when it does occur it is important to identify characteristics in the patients which may lead to further knowledge of the cause of the atherosclerosis, not only in this group but in general. As discussed in another chapter of this book there is an increased frequency of ischaemic heart disease in women taking oral contraceptives. As the use of these drugs is now so common in younger women it is only the relatively older studies that can attempt to identify inherent characteristics of young women with ischaemic heart disease. Few studies have specifically investigated the youngest women with atherosclerosis, and coronary artery disease is the only clinical complication of atherosclerosis which occurs in great enough numbers for valid study.

In a study of 146 women, average age of myocardial infarction 64 years, there was a sharp upswing in the frequency of myocardial infarction after the age of 45 and the average age of menopause of these women was 47.4 years[16]. There was a high incidence of diabetes (9.4%) and hypertension (48.6%) or both (11.6%) in younger women with myocardial infarction. Only one pre-menopausal woman had a myocardial infarction without having any other identifiable risk factors for the disease. In a large Scandinavian study[6] of women under the age of 60 with myocardial infarction, those who had myocardial infarctions had higher triglyceride levels but no difference in cholesterol; more hypertension; a higher prevalence of smoking; and those who smoked, smoked more; and more diabetes, compared to women of the same age who had not had myocardial infarction. The women with myocardial infarction undertook less physical activity than the controls and premature menopause was more common. Multiple risk factors were common. When women and men aged 50–54 without myocardial infarction were compared for risk factors for heart disease, men smoked more and consumed more alcohol, but there was no other difference in risk factors. The conclusion was that younger women who develop myocardial infarction very often have other identifiable risk factors for the disease. However, it was felt that the sex difference in the incidence of myocardial infarction could only be partially explained by the difference in frequency of known risk factors. In a British survey of ischaemic heart disease in young women[17] 46% of the women who had had a myocardial infarction had serum cholesterol of 270 mg% or more, 34% had a diastolic blood pressure of 100 mmHg or more and 32% smoked more than 20 cigarettes per day. Overall 74% had one or more risk factors. In addition 20% had had a premature menopause, 8% were on oral contraceptives, 5% were more than 15% overweight, 5% had diabetes or abnormal glucose tolerance tests, and 78% had abnormal blood lipid levels, most commonly raised serum cholesterol. Only 11% of these young women with ischaemic heart disease had no identifiable risk factors. Another British study[18] looked at 77 women with myocardial infarction and 207 controls, all aged less than 45 years of age. Women with myocardial infarction differed from controls in the number of cigarettes they smoked; the frequency of hypercholesterolaemia; and having had treatment for pretoxaemia, hypertension or diabetes. Obesity and a history of psychiatric illness were not independently associated with myocardial infarction. Overall 81.1% of the myocardial infarction patients had identifiable risk factors for atherosclerosis compared to 36% of the controls. In 24 young women aged 40 or less who had a clinical diagnosis of myocardial infarction, 20 had atherosclerosis and of these 4 had diabetes, 7 increased cholesterol, 1 increased blood pressure and 7 were on oral contraceptives[19]. Virtually all the women had risk factors for coronary artery disease.

Overall, therefore, ischaemic heart disease in young women is rare and when it does occur it is usually associated with known risk factors for atherosclerosis. The high frequency of risk factors for atherosclerosis in young women with ischaemic heart disease is particularly striking when compared with the levels of these factors, particularly lipids and lipoproteins, in women of the same age in the general community[20–22]. The high frequency of risk factors in young women with ischaemic heart disease is evidence in favour of a pathogenetic role for these factors and suggests that they overcome an inherent resistance to atherosclerosis in younger women. On the other hand, the resistance to atherosclerosis in young women is not entirely due to a lower prevalence of risk factors.

MENOPAUSE AND CORONARY HEART DISEASE

As the incidence of coronary heart disease increases with age in women and tends to become equal to that in men in older ages, it has been suggested that the changes associated with the menopause may be related to atherosclerosis. The high frequency of post-menopausal women among those with premature coronary artery disease has already been quoted.

The strongest evidence of a relationship of the menopause to coronary artery disease has come from the Framingham study, in which 2873 women were followed for more than 20 years. Compared with men, women had a degree of immunity from myocardial infarction, but this did not apply to angina pectoris or cerebrovascular disease[4]. The only condition in which the incidence of ischaemic heart disease was the same in women and in men at all ages was diabetes mellitus[23]. The presence of cardiovascular risk factors determined whether a woman would be at high or low risk for atherosclerosis within her sex, but did not explain the difference between males and females in the frequency of the disease[4]. The menopause was associated with a rise in serum cholesterol but no effect on blood pressure, blood glucose or body weight[24]. After 24 years follow-up no premenopausal women had developed myocardial infarction or died of coronary heart disease[25]. The risk of coronary heart disease in premenopausal women compared to men was 1 : 15 and most premenopausal heart disease was angina pectoris (Table 9.3). The risk of coronary heart disease in women who had had a surgical menopause was 2.7 times the risk in premenopausal women. A surgical menopause conferred a higher risk than a natural menopause and the risk was not related to cigarette smoking. The data from the Framingham study suggest that the impact of the menopause is substantial, relatively abrupt, and augments afterwards slowly, if at all[25]. Conversely, premature menopause was much more common in women with ischaemic heart disease than in women of the same age in the general population[26] (Table 9.4). In this study postmenopausal women had higher

Table 9.3 Coronary heart disease incidence for women in relation to the menopause (cases per 1000 per year) (the Framingham study[25])

Age (years)	Pre-	Post-	Ratio
Natural menopause			
40–44	0.2	0	–
45–49	1.2	3.4	2.8
50–54	1.7	4.4	2.6
Surgical menopause			
40–44	0.2	3.6	18
45–49	1.2	3.0	2.5
50–54	1.7	4.5	2.6

Table 9.4 Women who had the menopause at age 45 or less in two studies, and who had myocardial infarction or angina pectoris, compared with women in a population sample of the same age (percentage)[26]

	Women with ischaemic heart disease	Reference group of women
Case control study	20	12
Prospective study	35	12

serum cholesterol and triglycerides and were more likely to smoke cigarettes than premenopausal women, but they had lower blood pressures.

The suggestion that the menopause has a substantial and abrupt impact on coronary heart disease in women is not supported by mortality statistics from most countries. These indicate that the mortality from ischaemic heart disease in women steadily increases and that no sharp rise occurs at about the menopausal age. Furthermore, the conclusions drawn from the Framingham study are based on very small numbers of subjects[27].

Other studies, some of them cross-sectional, have looked at the effect of the menopause on some risk factors for atherosclerosis. However, the reports have not agreed on the effects of the menopause on cholesterol[28,29], triglyceride[28], blood pressure[28,30], and body weight[29]. Analysis of data in pre- and postmenopausal women is difficult[31]. Thus as the number of postmenopausal women increases the number of premenopausal women decreases. This occurs with advancing age, which is itself associated with an increase in atherosclerosis. Another problem is that the relative immunity of young women does not appear to apply to American black women who have a much higher death rate than white women from atherosclerotic heart disease. The reasons for this are not clear. A further problem is that the sex difference in ischaemic heart disease seems to depend on the type of clinical presentation. Myocardial infarction and sudden death are considerably more common in young men than young women. On the other hand, angina pectoris and ECG changes do not show the same difference[32].

HORMONAL CHANGES IN RELATION TO ATHEROSCLEROSIS AND THE MENOPAUSE

The main changes that occur after the menopause[33,34] are decreases in the ovarian secretion of oestrone and oestradiol, progesterone, androstenedione, dehydroepiandrosterone and a smaller decrease in testosterone. Before the menopause circulating oestradiol levels are greater than oestrone but the reverse is true after the menopause. Although oestrone secretion from the ovary decreases, some is still secreted by the adrenal and the percentage conversion of androstenedione to oestrone increases. The amount of oestrone produced by extraglandular tissue may actually be increased in premenopausal women and as body fat appears to be responsible for part of this conversion[35], obesity may be associated with relatively high levels of this hormone. Thus, in most postmenopausal women the major circulating oestrogen is oestrone which arises by extraglandular conversion of androstenedione. Although the post-menopausal ovary continues to secrete small quantities of testosterone and androstenedione, the adrenal is the predominant source of sex hormone production in postmenopausal women.

ARTIFICIAL MENOPAUSE AND CORONARY HEART DISEASE

There have been a number of studies on the effect of surgically induced menopause on the incidence of coronary artery disease and the results conflict. In general the older studies suggest an increased prevalence of ischaemic heart disease after an artificial menopause but more recent studies do not confirm this.

In an autopsy study atherosclerosis was more extensive in women who had had ovariectomy than in age-matched control women but less than in men of the same age[36]. Severe atherosclerosis was 45% greater in women who had had the operation and the main site of the disease was in the anterior descending branch of the left coronary artery. Another autopsy study[37] investigated the time interval between ovariectomy under the age of 50 years and the development of excessive coronary atherosclerosis. Patients on hormone therapy or who had diabetes were excluded. All women who had had the operation, and those who had had the operation more than 10 years beforehand, showed an increased incidence of coronary heart disease. However, excess atherosclerosis did not become evident until about 14 years after the operation.

In 102 women who had had bilateral ovariectomy under the age of 45, none of whom was taking oestrogen replacement therapy, premature menopause was associated with an increased incidence of clinical atherosclerosis including coronary heart disease[38]. This was not influenced by the presence of diabetes or hypertension. In a later study women who had had bilateral ovariectomy at less than 45 years of age were compared with women who had had hysterectomy alone at the same age[39]. None of the subjects was on hormone replacement therapy. Total cardiovascular disease in subjects who had had ovariectomy was 26.5% compared to 4.4% in those who had not had this operation. The type of cardiovascular disease was mainly angina pectoris. Similarly, bilateral ovariectomy was associated with an increase in the incidence of coronary artery disease and a rise in serum cholesterol levels[40]. Unilateral ovariectomy had no such effect. Thirty-five women who had menopause under the age of 40 had seven times the rate of coronary heart disease compared to women who had the menopause later[41]. Cholesterol and triglyceride were higher with premature menopause and increased with the length of time since the menopause. However, it took at least 10 years from the menopause for the development of ischaemic heart disease to become apparent.

Other studies have come to different conclusions. An autopsy study[42] examined 85 women who had had bilateral ovariectomy and 250 controls. None of the subjects was on hormone therapy and no difference in the extent of atherosclerosis was found between the subjects and controls. A similar conclusion was made in a study using angiography[43]. Twenty women aged less than 50 years who had had bilateral ovariectomy at least 5 years beforehand were compared with 65 controls of the same age. Five of the 20 operated women, and 23 of the 65 controls, had coronary artery disease on coronary angiography. There was no difference in risk factors for atherosclerosis, including serum cholesterol and glucose tolerance, between those who had had the operation and those who had not. Another study[44] of 104 women with myocardial infarction showed no correlation between the date of the menopause, whether early or late, natural or artificial, and the age at which myocardial infarction occurred.

Thus, the evidence on the effect of surgical menopause on the incidence of atherosclerosis remains contradictory. A review of the evidence[45] has set out a number of criteria which need to be followed before published studies can be considered to provide convincing evidence of a connection between bilateral ovariectomy and premature cardiovascular disease. The authors found that none of the evidence entirely fulfilled the criteria and they found the published data unconvincing. A connection between premature surgically induced menopause and cardiovascular disease in women remains unproven.

MALE SEX AND CORONARY HEART DISEASE

An alternative to the idea that younger women are protected from coronary heart disease is that there is a factor in men that promotes the disease[46]. An analysis of the death rates by age in men and women suggests that there is a curvilinear relationship between age and death rate and that this can be resolved into two straight lines. The break in the two lines, in both males and females, occurs at about age 50. Up to that age the slope of death rate against age is similar in both sexes but over the age of 50 the slope is less in men, suggesting that the rate of increase in mortality from coronary heart disease decreases after the age of 50 in men more than in women. It was suggested therefore, that rather than women losing a protective effect against atherosclerosis at around the age of 50, that men lose a promoting factor. The nature of this promoting factor remains unclear. The interpretation of these results is directly opposite to the suggestion of an increased risk in women which occurs at about the time of the menopause. This increase in risk in women, as described in the Framingham studies, was an absolute risk and was not related to incidence rates in men of the same age.

Sex hormone secretion in men also changes at around the age of 50. In 154 adult males aged between 20 and 90 total and free testosterone levels remained unchanged from the age of 20 to 50 and then fell progressively[47]. Mean levels were very low after the age of 70 although some very old men had levels which were as high as those in younger men. A further study from the same laboratory[48] found that compared to men aged less than 50, men aged more than 65 had increased levels of oestradiol, oestrone, LH and FSH. The testosterone levels were lower in the older men so that the testosterone : oestradiol ratio fell. Free testosterone levels were particularly depressed in the older men, and free oestradiol levels slightly increased resulting in a considerable increase in the ratios of free oestradiol to free testosterone. Other laboratories have confirmed the fall in testosterone with a rise[49] or no change[50] in oestradiol, and a pronounced fall in the testosterone : oestradiol ratio with increasing age. LH and FSH levels also rise, presumably related to lack of feedback inhibition of secretion by falling testosterone levels[50]. All studies agree that the changes start to become evident in men aged between 40 and 50 years.

There is thus a statistical suggestion that the male sex may promote ischaemic heart disease in young men and that the promoting factor loses its power after the age of 50. Coincident with this are hormonal changes causing a fall in the ratio of testosterone to oestradiol. Whether there is any direct relation between the hormone changes and the changing prevalence of ischaemic heart disease is unknown.

SEX HORMONE LEVELS IN MYOCARDIAL INFARCTION

There have been no published studies of sex hormone levels in relation to ischaemic heart disease in females. However, a study of 15 men aged between 32 and 42 who had had myocardial infarction indicated a high prevalence of feminizing features such as slow beard growth or gynaecomastia which preceded the myocardial infarction[8]. None of the subjects had hyperlipidaemia, diabetes, hypertension or smoked. Oestradiol and oestrone levels, measured at least 4 months after the infarction, were elevated compared to men of the same age who did not have heart disease, while the testosterone and dihydrotestosterone levels were unchanged (Table 9.5). In a further study[51] of the same men, which included measurements of glucose tolerance and serum lipids, it was found that the oestrogen : testosterone (E : T) ratio discriminated best between men with myocardial infarction and controls. The E : T ratio was found to correlate positively with the total glucose response to a glucose tolerance

Table 9.5 Plasma oestrogens and androgens and oestradiol : testosterone ratio (E : T) in young men with myocardial infarction, and in controls[8]

	Ischaemic heart disease (n = 15)	Controls (n = 15)	p
Age (years)	39.5 ± 3.1	38.8 ± 3.4	
Oestradiol (pg/ml)	43.5 ± 8.8	33.3 ± 5.5	<0.001
Oestrone (pg/ml)	50.7 ± 9.5	37.5 ± 5.8	<0.001
Testosterone (ng/ml)	7.68 ± 2.27	6.78 ± 1.57	N.S.
Dihydrotestosterone (ng/ml)	1.02 ± 0.24	0.93 ± 0.20	N.S.
E : T	5.7	4.9	

test, the total insulin response and the ratio of the insulin and glucose responses. Serum cholesterol also correlated with the E : T ratio while triglyceride correlated with the glucose area, the insulin : glucose ratio and cholesterol. It was suggested that lipid and carbohydrate abnormalities are important in the pathogenesis of atherosclerosis but that these are secondary to abnormalities in sex hormone secretion[51]. Two other studies of young male survivors of myocardial infarction have shown similar abnormalities of sex hormone levels but a further study of ischaemic heart disease and a study of stroke survivors have not confirmed these findings. A

Scottish study found high oestradiol and oestrone levels but normal testosterone and androstenedione levels[9] while an American study, reported only in abstract form[52], of 18 males with ischaemic heart disease 10 of whom had acute myocardial infarction and 63 normal controls, found that oestradiol was higher in those with ischaemic heart disease, particularly if they had complications, but testosterone and oestrone levels were unchanged. LH levels were lower in the men with ischaemic heart disease. A recent British study[53] has identified the effects of drugs, particularly clofibrate, on testosterone levels. When the effects of drugs were taken into account there were no significant differences in testosterone, oestrone and oestradiol levels between subjects with ischaemic heart disease and controls. Another factor often associated with ischaemic heart disease which influences sex hormone levels is smoking, which may cause raised oestrogen levels[54]. Obesity is also associated with both coronary disease and changes in sex hormone levels[35] and has not been taken into account in these studies.

In contrast to the findings in ischaemic heart disease, there were no abnormalities in sex hormone levels in young male survivors of stroke[10]. The subjects were 26 male survivors of stroke aged 46–64 years and they were compared with 27 healthy controls aged 45–64 years. None of the subjects had evidence of ischaemic heart disease and the stroke subjects had clinical evidence of a completed stroke at least 3 months prior to the study. Drugs affecting hormone status and smoking were taken into account. No difference was found in the oestradiol and testosterone levels nor in the E : T ratio between the stroke subjects and controls (Table 9.6).

Table 9.6 Plasma oestradiol and testosterone levels and oestradiol : testosterone ratio (E : T) in young men with strokes, and in controls[10]

	Strokes (n = 25)	Controls (n = 27)
Age (years)	56	57
Oestradiol (pmol/l)	96 ± 9.4	96 ± 8.0
Testosterone (nmol/l)	11.1 ± 1.0	11.0 ± 0.6
E : T	10.0 ± 1.2	9.7 ± 1.0

A number of possible reasons for the different results in stroke and ischaemic heart disease are possible. One is that the age of the stroke subjects was somewhat higher and the association of oestrogen and vascular disease may only occur in the younger age groups. It may be that the pathogenesis of stroke is different from that of myocardial infarction. However, the same stroke subjects had a similar pattern of HDL levels to that found in myocardial infarction[55]. It is possible that the abnormal oestrogen levels are associated with heart disease rather than with atherosclerosis. An investigation of sex hormone levels in subjects with proven atherosclerosis but not infarction is needed to answer this question.

Whatever the explanation, none of the studies provides evidence of a protective effect of oestrogens against atherosclerosis and they tentatively suggest a harmful association of oestrogen and heart disease. However, the inconsistencies in the results and the recently discovered confounding effects of drugs and smoking make further well-controlled studies essential before any conclusions can be drawn on the relationship of endogenous sex hormone secretion and atherosclerosis.

CONCLUSIONS

It can be accepted that myocardial infarction is commoner in young men than young women in areas where the incidence of ischaemic heart disease is high. There is also agreement that the majority of young women who develop ischaemic heart disease have identifiable risk factors for atherosclerosis. The differential sex incidence for myocardial infarction does not apply to cerebrovascular disease and does not occur in areas where the general incidence of ischaemic heart disease is low. This suggests that there is a factor or factors which specifically promotes cardiac ischaemia, presumably due to coronary atherosclerosis in men, in developed parts of the world, and which does not affect the cerebral arterial system. While risk factors for atherosclerosis are more common in young men than young women this does not entirely explain the sex difference in heart disease.

In later life the sex difference in incidence of ischaemic heart disease tends to disappear. There is no agreement on whether this is caused by the loss of a protective effect in young women or the loss of a promoting effect in young men (or possibly both). Similarly, the effect of the menopause on ischaemic heart disease is not clear. It is difficult to reconcile a rise in myocardial infarctions after the menopause with no effect on angina pectoris. It is also difficult to reconcile the findings of an abrupt effect of the menopause on myocardial infarction in epidemiological studies with the steady rise in prevalence found in national mortality statistics. The relationship of changes in ischaemic heart disease incidence at the menopause to lipid disorders and smoking habits is worthy of further study.

Changes in hormone secretion, particularly in the ratio of oestrogens to androgens, in ageing men and women are obvious candidates for an explanation of the sex differences in ischaemic heart disease. However, there is no clear pathogenic role for these hormones in the development of atherosclerosis. While a reduction in oestrogen levels in postmenopausal women might be related to the apparent loss of protection against coronary artery disease, there are inconsistent reports of high oestrogen levels in men with myocardial infarction. Further well-controlled studies of sex hormone levels in the different clinical syndromes of atherosclerosis in men and women are urgently needed.

The role of endogenous sex hormone secretion on atherosclerosis is far from clear. The remaining chapters in this section will discuss the effects of exogenous sex hormones on atherosclerosis and lipid metabolism, and the effects of sex hormones on experimental vascular disease.

References

1. Oliver, M. F. (ed.) (1978). *Coronary Heart Disease in Young Women.* (Edinburgh: Churchill Livingstone)
2. Editorial (1977). Coronary heart disease in young women. *Lancet,* **2,** 282
3. Kagan, A., Dawber, T. R., Kannel, W. B. and Revotskie, N. (1962). The Framingham study: a prospective study of coronary heart diseases. *Fed. Proc.,* **21,** suppl. 2, 52
4. Kannel, W. B., Hjortland, M. C., McNamara, P. M. and Gordon, T. (1976). Menopause and risk of cardiovascular disease. The Framingham study. *Ann. Intern. Med.,* **85,** 447
5. Kannel, W. B., Dawber, T. R., Cohen, M. E. and McNamara, P. M. (1965). Vascular disease of the brain – epidemiologic aspects: The Framingham study. *Am. J. Publ. Health,* **55,** 1355
6. Bengtsson, C. (1973). Ischaemic heart disease in women. *Acta Med. Scand.,* suppl. 549, 1
7. Haberman, S., Capildeo, R. and Rose, F. C. (1978). The changing mortality of cerebrovascular disease. *Q. J. Med.,* **47,** 71
8. Phillips, G. B. (1976). Evidence for hyperoestrogenaemia as a risk factor for myocardial infarction in men. *Lancet,* **2,** 14
9. Entrican, J. G., Beach, C., Carroll, D. *et al.* (1978). Raised plasma oestradiol and oestrone levels in young survivors of myocardial infarction. *Lancet,* **2,** 487
10. Taggart, H., Sheridan, B. and Stout, R. W. (1980). Sex hormone levels in younger male stroke survivors. *Atherosclerosis,* **35,** 123
11. Goodale, F., Thomas, W. A. and O'Neal, R. M. (1960). Myocardial infarction in women. *Arch. Pathol.,* **69,** 599
12. Mitchell, J. R. A. and Schwartz, C. J. (1965). *Arterial Disease.* (Oxford: Blackwell)
13. Kuller, L. and Lilienfeld, A. (1966). Epidemiological study of sudden and unexpected deaths due to arteriosclerotic heart disease. *Circulation,* **34,** 1056
14. Sternley, N. H. (1968). Atherosclerosis in a defined population. *Acta Pathol. Microbiol. Scand.,* suppl. **194,** 1
15. Tejada, C., Strong, J. P., Montenegro, M. R., Restrepo, C. and Selberg, L. A. (1968). Distribution of coronary and aortic atherosclerosis by geographic location, race and sex. *Lab. Invest.,* **18,** 509
16. James, J. N., Post, H. W. and Smith, F. J. (1955). Myocardial infarction in women. *Ann. Intern. Med.,* **43,** 153
17. Oliver, M. F. (1974). Ischaemic heart disease in young women. *Br. Med. J.,* **4,** 253
18. Mann, J. I., Doll, R., Thorogood, M., Vessey, M. P. and Waters, W. E. (1976). Risk factors for myocardial infarction in young women. *Br. J. Prev. Soc. Med.,* **30,** 94
19. Morris, D. C., Hurst, J. W. and Logue, R. B. (1976). Myocardial infarction in young women. *Am. J. Cardiol.,* **38,** 299
20. Adlersberg, D., Schaefer, L. E., Steinberg, A. G. and Wang, C. I. (1956). Age, sex, serum lipids and coronary atherosclerosis. *J. Am. Med. Assoc.,* **162,** 619
21. Wood, P. D. S., Stern, M. P. and Silvers, A. (1972). Prevalence of plasma lipoprotein abnormalities in a free-living population of the Central Valley, California. *Circulation,* **45,** 114
22. Lewis, B., Chait, A., Wooton, I. D. P. *et al.* (1974). Frequency of risk factors for ischaemic heart disease in a healthy British population. *Lancet,* **1,** 141
23 Garcia, M. J., McNamara, P. M., Gordon, T. and Kannel, W. B. (1974). Morbidity and mortality in diabetics in the Framingham population. Sixteen year follow-up study. *Diabetes,* **23,** 105
24. Hjortland, M. C., McNamara, P. M. and Kannel, W. B. (1976). Some atherogenic concomitants of menopause: the Framingham study. *Am. J. Epidemiol.,* **103,** 304
25. Gordon, T., Kannel, W. B., Hjortland, M. C. and McNamara, P. M. (1978). Menopause and coronary heart disease. The Framingham study. *Ann. Intern. Med.,* **89,** 157

110 HORMONES AND ATHEROSCLEROSIS

26. Bengtsson, A. and Lindquist, O. (1978). Coronary heart disease during the menopause. In Oliver, M. F. (ed.) *Coronary Heart Disease in Young Women*, pp. 234–42. (Edinburgh: Churchill Livingstone)
27. Editorial (1977). Coronary heart disease and the menopause. *Br. Med. J.*, **1**, 862
28. Weiss, N. S. (1972). Relationship of menopause to serum cholesterol and arterial blood pressure – the United States health examination survey of adults. *Am. J. Epidemiol.*, **96**, 237
29. Hallberg, L. and Svanborg, A. (1967). Cholesterol, phospholipids and triglycerides in plasma in 50 year-old women. *Acta Med. Scand.*, **181**, 185
30. Taylor, R. D., Corcoron, A. C. and Page, I. H. (1974). Menopausal hypertension: a critical study. *Am. J. Med. Sci.*, **213**, 475
31. Doll, R. (1978). Discussion. In Oliver, M. F. (ed.) *Coronary Heart Disease in Young Women*, pp. 22–3. (Edinburgh: Churchill Livingstone)
32. Wilhelmsen, L. (1978). Epidemiology of coronary heart disease in young women. In Oliver, M. F. (ed.) *Coronary Heart Disease in Young Women*, pp. 3–9. (Edinburgh: Churchill Livingstone)
33. Baird, D. T. (1978). Patterns of sex hormone production in women. In Oliver, M. F. (ed.) *Coronary Heart Disease in Young Women*, pp. 95–100. (Edinburgh: Churchill Livingstone)
34. Vermeulen, A. (1978). Patterns of sex hormone production in men. In Oliver, M. F. (ed.) *Coronary Heart Disease in Young Women*, pp. 101–5. (Edinburgh: Churchill Livingstone)
35. Kley, H. K., Edelmann, P. and Kruskemper, H. L. (1980). Relationship of plasma sex hormones to different parameters of obesity in male subjects. *Metabolism*, **29**, 1041
36. Wuest, J. E., Dry, T. J. and Edwards, J. E. (1953). The degree of coronary atherosclerosis in bilaterally oophorectomised women. *Circulation*, **7**, 801
37. Parrish, H. M., Carr, C. A., Hall, D. G. and King, T. M. (1967). Time interval from castration in premenopausal women to development of excessive coronary atherosclerosis. *Am. J. Obstet. Gynecol.*, **99**, 155
38. Robinson, R. W., Higano, N. and Cohen, W. D. (1959). Increased incidence of coronary heart disease in women castrated prior to the menopause. *Arch. Intern. Med.*, **104**, 908
39. Higano, N., Robinson, R. W. and Cohen, W. D. (1963). Increased incidence of cardiovascular disease in castrated women: two year follow-up study. *N. Engl. J. Med.*, **268**, 1123
40. Oliver, M. F. and Boyd, G. S. (1959). Effect of bilateral ovariectomy on coronary-artery disease and serum-lipid levels. *Lancet*, **2**, 690
41. Sznajderman, M. and Oliver, M. F. (1963). Spontaneous premature menopause, ischaemic heart disease and serum lipids. *Lancet*, **1**, 962.
42. Novak, E. R. and Williams, T. J. (1960). Autopsy comparison of cardiovascular changes in castrated and normal women. *Am. J. Obstet. Gynecol.*, **80**, 863
43. Manchester, J. H., Herman, M. V. and Gorlin, R. (1971). Premenopausal castration and documented coronary atherosclerosis. *Am. J. Cardiol.*, **28**, 33
44. Blanc, J. J., Boschat, J., Morin, I.-F., Clavier, J. and Penther, T. (1977). Menopause and myocardial infarction. *Am. J. Obstet. Gynecol.*, **127**, 353
45. Roberts, W. C. and Giraldo, A. A. (1979). Bilateral oophorectomy in menstruating women and accelerated coronary atherosclerosis: an unproved connection. *Am. J. Med.*, **67**, 363
46. Heller, R. F. and Jacobs, H. S. (1978). Coronary heart disease in relation to age, sex and the menopause. *Br. Med. J.*, **1**, 472
47. Vermeulen, A., Rubens, R. and Verdonck, L. (1972). Testosterone secretion and metabolism in male senescence. *J. Clin. Endocrinol. Metab.*, **34**, 730
48. Rubens, R., Dhont, M. and Vermeulen, A. (1974). Further studies on Leydig cell function in old age. *J. Clin. Endocrinol. Metab.*, **39**, 40
49. Pirke, K. M. and Doerr, P. (1973). Age-related changes and interrelationships between plasma testosterone, oestradiol and testosterone-oestradiol binding globulin in normal adult males. *Acta Endocrinol.*, **74**, 792
50. Stearns, E. L., MacDonnell, J. A., Kaufman, B. J. *et al.* (1974). Declining testicular function with age. Hormonal and clinical correlates. *Am. J. Med.*, **57**, 761
51. Phillips, G. B. (1977). Relationship between serum sex hormones and glucose, insulin,

and lipid abnormalities in men with myocardial infarction. *Proc. Natl. Acad. Sci. USA*, **74**, 1729

52. Levin, L. C. and Koreman, S. G. (1978). Elevated estradiol levels in acute MI and coronary artery disease. *Clin. Res.*, **26**, 308A
53. Heller, R. F., Jacobs, H. S., Vermeulen, A. and Deslypere, J. P. (1981). Androgens, oestrogens and coronary heart disease. *Br. Med. J.*, **282**, 438
54. Carr, D. (1978). Oestrogens, myocardial infarction and smoking. *Lancet*, **2**, 1048
55. Taggart, H. and Stout, R. W. (1979). Reduced high density lipoprotein in stroke: relationship with elevated triglyceride and hypertension *Eur. J. Clin. Invest.*, **9**, 219

10
Oestrogens, progestogens and cardiovascular disease

Oestrogens are prescribed to women in two circumstances – as part of oral contraceptive preparations, or as postmenopausal hormone replacement therapy. Oestrogens may also be prescribed to men as part of the treatment of prostatic carcinoma or to lower plasma cholesterol. The relationship of oestrogens and, in the case of oral contraceptives, progestogens to cardiovascular disease has been studied in all these circumstances. This chapter will review the evidence of a relationship between these sex hormones and disease of the coronary or cerebral arteries. Oestrogens are also associated with venous thromboembolism but this will not be discussed here.

ORAL CONTRACEPTIVES AND CARDIOVASCULAR DISEASE

Evidence on the association of oestrogens and cardiovascular disease comes from reports of adverse effects of oral contraceptives in younger women. The major epidemiological tools used in studying the relationship of contraceptives and cardiovascular disease have been retrospective or case control studies and prospective or cohort studies[1]. Different types of information are obtained from these two types of studies and the results are reported in different ways. Two common terms are relative risk, which is the ratio of the incidence of a disease among drug users to that of non-users, and attributable risk, which is the difference in the incidence of a disease between drug users and non-users. The latter better conveys the clinical importance of the effect of a drug on the occurrence of a disease.

The earliest reports were concerned with increased frequency of thromboembolic phenomena, including deep venous thrombosis and pulmonary embolism. Venous thromboembolic disease has an increased incidence in oral contraceptive users[1]. The effect appears to be primarily due to the oestrogen component of the drugs, involves decreased antithrombolytic activity and is probably exacerbated in women who do not have an appropriate increase in fibrinolytic activity in response to increased intravenous clotting. However, later case control and cohort studies reported that the use of oral contraceptives is also associated with an increase in the frequency of strokes and myocardial infarction[2] (Table 10.1). Although a high frequency of oral contraceptive use in young women with myocardial infarction had been noted earlier[3] the first evidence of an association of oral contraceptives with myocardial infarction from studies specifically designed to test this question came in a series of reports in 1975.

Table 10.1   Studies of oral contraceptive use and cardiovascular disease

Author	End-point	Relative risk (users per non-user)
Collaborative Group, 1973[19]	stroke	9.0
Mann et al., 1975[4]	MI survivor	4.5
		age 30–39, 2.7
		age 40–44, 5.7
Mann and Inman, 1975[6]	MI death	age 30–39, 2.8
		age 40–44, 4.7
Mann et al., 1975[5]	MI	3.1
Mann et al., 1976[7]	MI death	age 40–44, 3.0
Shapiro et al., 1979[8]	MI	4.0
Jick et al., 1978[9]	MI non-fatal	15.0
Pettiti et al., 1979[10]	SAH fatal	6.0
Krueger et al., 1980[12]	MI (white women only)	4.0
Slone et al., 1981[17]	MI	3.5

MI = myocardial infarction
SAH = subarachnoid haemorrhage

A case control study of female survivors of myocardial infarction less than 45 years of age[4,5] found that 29.3% of the young women with myocardial infarction had used oral contraceptives within a month of the illness, compared to 8.4% of the controls. There was no difference in the menopausal status in the myocardial infarction subjects and the controls. Other associations with myocardial infarction included cigarette smoking, hypertension, diabetes, obesity and raised plasma cholesterol and triglyceride. There was a suggestion that oral contraceptives interacted with smoking to greatly increase the risk of myocardial infarction, and that the risk factors were synergistic. In a retrospective mortality survey, in which death certificates were used to identify younger women who had died from myocardial infarction, and in which drug usage was ascertained from general practitioners, it was found that in women who used oral contraceptives, the risk of death from myocardial infarction was increased by 2.8-fold in those aged 30–39 and by 4.7-fold in those aged 40–44[6]. The risk was related to the duration of use, current users being particularly at risk, but was not related to the dose of oestrogen in the preparation. There was no difference in the frequency of premature menopause in the two groups. Although hypertension and diabetes were more common in those with myocardial infarction, the effect of oral contraceptives was independent of their effects. In this type of retrospective survey, smoking habits could not be accurately ascertained. There was a suggestion that mortality might be related more to intra-arterial thrombosis than to vessel wall disease as 83% of post-mortem reports in oral contraceptive users mentioned thrombosis in the coronary artery compared to 55% in non-users. However, this was not a planned randomized and blind control study of this point, and no more than a suggestion could be made. The apparent increased risk of older women was tested in a further retrospective analysis of the relationship of oral contraceptive use and fatal myocardial infarction in women aged 40–44[7]. Users of oral contraceptives in this age group had three times the risk of fatal myocardial infarction compared to non-users, and this effect was not influenced by a history of treatment for diabetes or hypertension.

Later studies confirmed the increased risk of myocardial infarction in oral contraceptive users[8,9] and the adverse effect of smoking[8]. However the studies did not all agree on whether previous use increased the risk[8]. A large American case control study[10] found no increase in risk of myocardial infarction in oral contraceptive users, but an increased risk of subarachnoid haemorrhage. The latter was confirmed by a large British study[11]. Another American case control study[12] carried out in the five largest metropolitan areas of the United States found an increased risk of myocardial infarction in women who did not have contraindications for using the pill.

The largest prospective study of the relation of oral contraceptives and cardiovascular disease is that of the Royal College of General Practitioners[11,13]. The study consists of over 23 000 women taking oral contraceptives, and an equal number of controls who have never taken the pill. Twice yearly reports on contraceptive use, morbidity and mortality are prepared by the patients' general practitioners. The latest report is based on 98 997 women-years of observation for current users of contraceptives, 84 811 for former users and 128 630 women-years for controls. Those who had ever used oral contraceptives had a 40% higher overall mortality rate than the controls and the excess risk was 23.3 per 100 000 women-years. The excess overall death rate was almost entirely due to the excess deaths from diseases of the circulatory system (Table 10.2). The major circulatory disorders which were associated with this excess risk were ischaemic heart disease and subarachnoid haemorrhage. Risks for strokes from other causes were very much smaller. Former users of the pill also had an excess risk of death, particularly from subarachnoid haemorrhage. The relative risk increased with increasing age for both smokers and non-smokers, and the relative risk was greater among smokers than among non-smokers for each age group. There was no relationship between the duration of oral contraceptive use and mortality.

Another large prospective study is the Oxford Family Planning

Table 10.2 Standardized mortality rate per 100 000 women-years by oral contraceptive use – Royal College of General Practitioners Study[11]

	Ever-users	Controls	Relative risk	Excess risk
All diseases of the circulatory system	29.9	7.2	4.2	22.7
Ischaemic heart disease	8.0	2.0	3.9	6.0
Subarachnoid haemorrhage	9.0	2.3	4.0	6.7
Stroke	5.7	2.7	2.1	3.0

Association Contraceptive study which is an investigation of 17 032 women aged 25–39 years attending 17 family planning clinics in England and Scotland[14]. Women taking oral contraceptives are compared with those using diaphragms or intrauterine devices. The characteristics of the subjects in the different groups are similar except that the oral contraceptive group smoke more than the others. By April 1977[15] 45 deaths had occurred. All nine deaths from cardiovascular disease involved women who were taking oral contraceptives. By 1981 there had been 79 678 women-years of observation of women on the pill and 62 532 women-years of observation in the other two groups which were combined and acted as controls[16]. Eighty-one deaths were included in the study. Of 13 deaths from circulatory disorders 10 were in women using oral contraceptives (Table 10.3). The authors consider that the data support the view that the pill is involved in the ætiology of myocardial infarction, especially in women who smoke. As only two of the women who had taken oral contraceptives were still taking the pill at the time of their deaths from myocardial infarction, the study suggests that there is a continuing increased risk in former users of the pill. No association of the pill with subarachnoid haemorrhage was found in this study.

Table 10.3 Standardized mortality ratios for circulatory disorders per 100 000 women-years in women using oral contraceptives and other methods of contraception (diaphragm or intrauterine device) – Oxford Family Planning Association Study[16]

Cause of death	Method of contraception	
	Oral	Others
All circulatory disorders	12.3	4.9
Ischaemic heart disease	9.7	1.7
Cerebrovascular disease	2.3	1.8

The studies reported so far have concerned the risk of myocardial infarction and stroke in patients currently taking oestrogen-containing preparations. The question as to whether the increased risk which has been demonstrated disappears when treatment is discontinued is also important. A hospital-based case control study has looked at this question[17]. In this study 556 women with myocardial infarction aged 25–49 years old were compared with 2036 age-matched control subjects. It was found that past users of oral contraceptives had an increased risk of myocardial infarction which was related to the duration of use of the preparations. For total duration of past use of less than 5 years, 5–9 years and 10 or more years respectively, the risk-ratio estimates were 1.0, 1.6 and 2.5 and the trend was statistically significant. For those without predisposing conditions, such as hypertension, diabetes or angina pectoris, the risk ratios were 1.1, 1.5 and 3.0 respectively with a statistically significant trend with increasing duration. The risks were nevertheless somewhat less than the 3.5 risk-ratio estimate for current users of the preparations. The increased risk with increased duration of use was found to be particularly strong in those aged 40–49 years. The data suggest that the risk of infarction is increased 2–3-fold in women who have used oral contraceptives for more than 10 years before discontinuation. The excess risk associated with long-term use occurred in subjects who had stopped taking contraceptives less than 5 years previously as well as in those who had stopped 5–9 years previously. The data was insufficient to assess whether stopping for more than 10 years had any influence. Unlike the reported results with current users of oral contraceptives the risk-ratio estimates declined with increasing cigarette smoking. The results of this study are significant with respect to hypotheses for the mechanism of the association of oral contraceptive use and myocardial infarction. It suggests that a more chronic pathological process than thrombosis is involved, and implicates atherosclerosis. This may be related to the effects of contraceptives on lipid metabolism, glucose tolerance and blood pressure but the long-term effect of the preparations on these complications was not recorded. This is the only large-scale report of this type and confirmation from other series is awaited.

A detailed study of the relationship of the dose of the oestrogen and progestogen components of oral contraception preparations to the risk of cardiovascular disease[18] found a significant association between the dose of both oestrogen and progestogen and the risk of death from ischaemic heart disease or stroke (Table 10.4). This was independent of the effect of these drugs on blood pressure. This suggests a direct effect of the preparations on the vascular system, but the mechanism of this remains unknown.

The evidence of an association between oral contraceptives and cardiovascular disease was reviewed in detail by Vessey in 1980[2] before publication of the latest results of the RCGP and Oxford studies. With regard to stroke, case control studies have provided strong evidence of a several-fold increase in the risk of thrombotic stroke in users of oral contraceptives. The data relating to haemorrhagic stroke are less convincing, although a slight increase in risk may exist. However, the findings with respect to stroke must be viewed with some caution in view of

Table 10.4 Effect of different doses of oestrogens or progestogens on the observed/expected (O : E) ratios of ischaemic heart disease and stroke

(a) Different doses of the oestrogen ethinyl oestradiol, 1974–77

	Ethinyloestradiol (μg)		
	30	50	p
Stroke O : E	0.82	1.20	n.s.
Ischaemic heart disease O : E	0.54	1.58	<0.01

(b) Different doses of the progestogen norethisterone acetate in preparations containing 50 μg ethinyl oestradiol, 1968–77

	Norethisterone acetate (mg)				
	1.0	2.5	3.0	4.0	p
Stroke O : E	0.75	0.69	1.12	1.39	<0.01
Ischaemic heart disease O : E	0.58	1.00	1.30	1.29	<0.001

(c) Different doses of the progestogen levonogestrel in preparations containing 30 μg ethinyl oestradiol, 1974–77

	Levonorgestrel (μg)		
	150	250	p
Stroke O : E	0.46	1.37	<0.05
Ischaemic heart disease O : E	1.40	0.67	n.s.

For differing doses of oestrogen or progestogen the other component of the contraceptive pill is constant (From Meade et al.[18])

the difficulty in making a clinical differentiation between the different types of stroke. Cohort studies have supported the results of the case control studies. There is some evidence that the risk of stroke may be positively correlated with the oestrogen content of oral contraceptives and there is also more recent evidence that the progestogen dose is also related to the risk of stroke. There is, however, no reliable evidence to show whether the risk of stroke is related to the duration of use of oral contraceptives. There is little evidence of any potentiation of the effects of oral contraceptives by other risk factors for stroke. With respect to myocardial infarction the evidence suggests a 2–4-fold increase in the risk of non-fatal myocardial infarction in users of oral contraceptives. Most of the evidence comes from case control studies but data from cohort studies support these findings. Myocardial infarction now appears to be the most important cardiovascular adverse effect of the contraceptive pill. The evidence relating the risk of myocardial infarction to the oestrogen content of oral contraceptives is inconclusive but there is evidence that the risk of arterial disease is positively correlated with progestogen content. Data suggesting a relationship between the duration of oral contraceptive use and myocardial infarction are sparse. There is evidence that risk factors for myocardial infarction may potentiate each other and be potentiated by the use of oral contraceptives. This is particularly the case for cigarette smoking. There is also evidence linking oral contraceptive use with venous thromboembolism and certain other types of vascular disease.

Pathological changes associated with oral contraceptives

There have been very few reports of autopsy studies of women taking oral contraceptives. The earliest study reported intimal thickening in the arteries[20]. Similar changes occur in many arteries in association with changes in female sex hormones in relation to pregnancy and parturition[21]. The exact nature of the cells involved in this proliferation was not clear but in other studies similar lesions show very active smooth muscle cells. Similar intimal thickening associated with proliferation of smooth muscle cells has been induced by ethinyl oestradiol in rats[22]. An alternative suggestion is that myocardial infarction in oral contraceptive users is due to oestrogens causing ulceration of pre-existing atheromatous plaques by removing lipid[23].

Oral contraceptives and blood pressure

A way in which oral contraceptives may be related to cardiovascular disease is by an effect on blood pressure. A prospective controlled study showed that after 4 years oral contraceptive use there was a mean rise in systolic blood pressure of 14.2 mmHg and in diastolic pressure of 8.5 mmHg[24]. This was related to the oestrogen dose and was unrelated to progestogens. A rise in blood pressure in women on oral contraceptives was also found in two community studies[25,26]. Hypertension is a risk factor for cardiovascular disease in women. A Swedish study[27] showed that angina pectoris and myocardial infarction were both increased in women with hypertension and there was the same relationship of hypertension to ischaemic heart disease in women as in men. The Framingham study also showed that the risk of coronary disease[28] and stroke[29] was related to hypertension in exactly the same way in women as in men although myocardial infarction was the commonest presentation in hypertensive men whereas angina pectoris was commonest in hypertensive women.

Oral contraceptives and clotting

Some reports have suggested that oral contraceptives might be associated with thrombosis rather than atherosclerosis[6]. This was supported by a coronary angiographic study of four young women who were on oral contraceptives and who had unequivocable evidence of myocardial infarction[30]. The coronary arteries were normal but myocardial perfusion was decreased in the area of the infarct. It was suggested that a thrombus or embolus had caused the infarct and that it had subsequently dissolved. Because of this a number of studies of the effect of oral contraceptives on various blood clotting mechanisms have been carried out. It has been found that platelet aggregation is increased by oral contraceptives in women[31,32], and by oestrogens in men[33]. Nevertheless there was no change in whole-blood clotting time or plasma recalcification time. Factor VI and factor X appeared to be increased, and this was due to the oestrogen, but not the progestogen[34]. The effect of oral contraceptives on blood clotting factors is greater when they contained 50 mg oestrogen than when they contained 30 mg oestrogen[35]. Alternatively it has been suggested that, rather than platelet changes, coagulation abnormalities and abnormalities in the fibrinolytic system may be responsible for the vascular disease[36]. It seems reasonable to conclude that oral contraceptives do alter various clotting mechanisms[37] but whether these are responsible for the undoubted increase in thrombosis that occurs is not clear. The correlation between *in vitro* tests of clotting and intravascular coagulation is not exact. Furthermore, tests of coagulation do not answer the question as to whether the increase in cardiovascular disease risk in users of oral contraceptives is entirely due to thrombosis *in situ* or whether vessel wall disease is the underlying process. It is possible that both processes occur, and indeed coagulation in the arterial wall may play a part in the pathogenesis of atherosclerosis.

OESTROGEN THERAPY AND CARDIOVASCULAR DISEASE

The relationship of sex hormones to atherosclerosis becomes even more confused when the association of non-contraceptive oestrogen therapy to cardiovascular disease is considered. The evidence can be reviewed under two headings: oestrogen therapy in postmenopausal women in whom the drugs are given to replace the decline in natural hormone secretion or to prevent postmenopausal oesteoporosis; and oestrogens given to men for treatment of prostatic carcinoma or in an attempt to prevent atherosclerosis.

Postmenopausal oestrogen therapy

There are relatively few studies of postmenopausal oestrogen therapy in relation to cardiovascular disease. The majority show no association but one suggests a beneficial effect and two a harmful effect (Table 10.5).

Among the studies which show no association is the Boston Collaborative Drugs Surveillance Program study[38] which found that in

Table 10.5   Studies of non-contraceptive oestrogen use and cardiovascular disease

Author	No. of Cases	Age (years)	End point	Relative risk (users per non-users)
Rosenberg et al., 1976[38]	336	40–75	MI	0.9
Pfeffer and van der Neort, 1976 [39]	210	58–98	stroke	1.1
Pfeffer et al., 1978[40]	220	44–100	MI	0.9
Gordon et al., 1978[44*]	25	40–54	CHD	1.6
Jick et al., 1978[45]	17	39–45	MI	7.5
Jick et al., 1978[46]	19	39–45	MI	9.3
Petitti et al., 1979[10]	not stated	18–54	MI	1.2
	not stated	18–54	SAH	1.6
	not stated	18–54	stroke	0.9
Hammond et al., 1979[50]	301	10–50	CHD	0.3
Rosenberg et al., 1980[41]	477	30–49	MI	1.0
Bain et al., 1981[42]	123	30–55	MI	0.9
Adam et al., 1981[43]	76	50–59	fatal MI	0.7
	23	50–59	fatal SAH	0.6
Ross et al., 1981[47]	133	mean 73	MI death	0.43

MI   = myocardial infarction
SAH = subarachnoid haemorrhage
CHD = coronary heart disease; i.e. angina pectoris, coronary insufficiency, myocardial infarction or cardiac death
* Cohort study; the remainder are case control studies

postmenopausal women aged 40–75 years of age, 4.9% of 6730 patients without ischaemic heart disease and 2.4% of 336 patients with myocardial infarction were users of oestrogen. The most common preparation used was premarin, a mixture of conjugated equine oestrogens. There was no evidence of a synergistic effect of oestrogen on other cardiovascular risk factors. After consideration of age, smoking, diabetes, hypertension and a past history of myocardial infarction, the risk-ratio of those taking oestrogen to those not was not different from one. Similar results were found in a case control study of oestrogen use and stroke in postmenopausal women in California[39]. Although there was highly significant association between hypertension diabetes and stroke, there was no association between oestrogen use and stroke. There was, however, a highly significant association between oestrogen use and a raised blood pressure. The dose of oestrogen used in these women was relatively small, much smaller than that used in men with prostatic carcinoma. A case control study[40] of women aged 57–98 years in the same southern California retirement community looked at the relation of myocardial infarction or angina pectoris to oestrogen treatment. The cases did not differ significantly from the controls with respect to age, body habitus, serum cholesterol, serum uric acid or blood pressure. Different measures of oestrogen use, including frequency of use, currency of use duration, and dose, were not significantly different among the cases and the controls. At some time during the study period, 30.1% of cases and 33.1% of controls had used oestrogens. Multiple discriminant analysis indicated that the single variable which best separated cases from controls was systolic blood pressure. Diabetic status added a further increment of separation. None of the discriminant function, multiple logistic or multiple regression analyses suggested that oestrogen dose or duration had any significant effect on coronary risk. The doses of oestrogen used by women in this study were again relatively small. The Walnut Creek Contraceptive Drug study[10] also found no effect of non-contraceptive oestrogens on myocardial infarction or subarachnoid haemorrhage. A case control study of the relationship of the use of non-contraceptive oestrogen and myocardial infarction in younger women[41] studied 477 women aged 30–49 years who had been admitted with an acute myocardial infarction. Control subjects were in-patients of the same hospital who had diseases other than myocardial infarction; 16% of the cases and 15% of the control subjects had used non-contraceptive oestrogens. Even when other influences such as smoking, hypertension, diabetes and abnormal blood lipids were taken into consideration, there was no evidence of an excess risk of myocardial infarction in those who had taken oestrogens. The majority of subjects who took oestrogens took conjugated oestrogens mostly in doses of 1.25 mg or less. The mean duration of oestrogen use was 33 months for the cases and 46 months for the control subjects.

A recent retrospective case control study[42] of 121 964 nurses aged 30–55 years compared the use of postmenopausal oestrogen replacement therapy in a group who had had non-fatal myocardial infarction and age-matched controls. Hormone use after the menopause was not appreciably different in the subjects who had myocardial infarction and the controls. Compared with women who had never used oestrogens the estimated risk of hospitalization from myocardial infarction was not significantly different from one. Adjusting for other risk factors including cigarette smoking, hypertension, diabetes and lipid levels did not alter this. The only exception was women who had had a bilateral oophorectomy who had a significantly decreased risk of myocardial infarction when on oestrogen replacement therapy. There has only been one British study[43] of the relationship of cardiovascular disease and hormone replacement treatment. This was a small pilot study using death certificates and case controls with prescribing and other information being obtained by postal questionnaire from general practitioners. The women who had died from acute myocardial infarction more often had a history of angina, previous acute myocardial infarction, stroke, diabetes, toxaemia, hypertension, hyperlipidemia and tobacco smoking than the controls. Hormone replacement therapy was uncommon in both groups of women, only 3% of both cases and controls receiving this treatment. There was little association between the presence of risk factors for myocardial infarction and the use of hormone replacement therapy, and the results provided no evidence of a change in the risk of cardiovascular disease in women receiving hormone replacement treatment. However, conclusions from this study are difficult as the numbers were small and hormone replacement was rarely used.

Two studies have found differences in the frequency of myocardial infarction in women using oestrogen therapy compared with controls. In the Framingham study[44] a rise in coronary heart disease incidence after the menopause was identified. Oestrogen use after the menopause was accompanied by a coronary heart disease incidence about twice that in women not receiving this treatment. A small study of women aged 39–45 years[45] found that 53% of 17 subjects with myocardial infarction gave a history of oestrogen use at the time of admission to hospital, compared with 12% of 34 age-matched controls. The most common oestrogen preparation used was conjugated oestrogen. As in other studies myocardial infarction in these young women was almost exclusively a disease of cigarette smokers. A later report of the same study[46] found an even greater difference – 53% of 19 women with myocardial infarction were non-contraceptive oestrogen users compared with 10% of controls. On the other hand, a case control study of older women in a Los Angeles retirement community[47] reported that ingestion of conjugated oestrogens, which was by far the most commonly used type of hormone replacement therapy, reduced the risk of death from ischaemic heart disease substantially and significantly. The beneficial effect was more apparent when other risk factors for ischaemic heart disease were absent and the association was not due to identifiable confounding factors. In those in whom the cause of death was confirmed by autopsy, the risk ratio was similar to those in whom autopsy had not been performed. Information was not obtained on the type of menopause nor the duration of oestrogen therapy.

The effect of oestrogens on plasma lipids and lipoproteins is discussed in Chapter 11. Reports differ, with some suggesting a reduction in plasma cholesterol[48,49] with little change in triglyceride, while others find no change in cholesterol and a rise in triglyceride[25]. There is similar disagreement on the effect of oestrogens on blood pressure[24,50] although all of the changes were small. The menopause results in a small increase in serum cholesterol and decrease in systolic blood pressure[51] and postmenopausal oestrogens do not completely reverse these changes.

It is difficult to draw conclusions from the published data on the relationship of postmenopausal oestrogen therapy to cardiovascular disease. The majority of case control studies, including the largest, find no association. On the other hand, the only cohort study in the series reported a harmful effect. The results of the studies on postmenopausal oestrogens and cardiovascular disease differ from those on contraceptive hormones where the risk of cardiovascular disease is increased, particularly in women who smoke. The reasons for the differences are not clear but may be related to the dose of oestrogen used in the different preparations. Doses tend to be higher in oral contraceptives. The type of oestrogen used is also different, contraceptives using synthetic hormones while conjugated natural oestrogens are most commonly used for postmenopausal replacement. The fact that oral contraceptives also contain a progestogen is also worthy of consideration, especially in view of the association between the dose of progestogen and the frequency of cardiovascular disease. The differences in endogenous oestrogen and progestogen secretion in pre- and postmenopausal women may also be a relevant factor. If, as is suggested in some reports, postmenopausal oestrogen therapy causes changes in plasma lipids and blood pressure which would tend to reduce the risk of atherosclerosis, oestrogens may have an effect on the artery which counteracts this benefit.

Oestrogen therapy in men

Because of the apparent beneficial effect of the female sex on cardiovascular disease, and because oestrogen therapy had been known to lower serum cholesterol, a number of trials of the effectiveness of oestrogen for preventing myocardial infarction in men have been carried out. In general the results of these trials have not shown benefit and in some the oestrogen therapy has had apparent deleterious effects.

The earliest studies of the influence of reduction of serum lipids on coronary heart disease used an oestrogen to lower cholesterol. Three trials, the reports of which were published in the early 1960s, produced differing results. In Edinburgh[52], 50 survivors of myocardial infarction were given 200 μg ethinyl oestradiol per day and were compared with 50 survivors who took a placebo. Although serum cholesterol was reduced by 18% and the cholesterol/phospholipid ratio by 28% in the oestrogen-treated groups, mortality and morbidity from myocardial infarction in the two groups were the same during the 5 years of the trial. In Chicago[53] 275 men under 50, all of whom had had a previous myocardial infarction at least 2 months before the start of the trial, were randomized into two groups. One group was given conjugated oestrogen at a starting dose of 1.25 mg/day rising to 10 mg/day. Early in the trial it was found that with the highest dose there was a very high incidence of cardiovascular disease, three-quarters of which was fatal. This dose was abandoned. Survival rates were 50% greater in those who had been on the lower doses of oestrogen for 5 years than those on a placebo preparation. No mention was made in the report of the effect of the hormone on serum lipid levels. Another early study[54] used 421 men who had had a myocardial infarction at least 3 months previously. Four different groups were used – two on different synthetic oestrogens, one on natural oestrogens and one on placebo. The 5-year survival for those on synthetic oestrogens was similar to that for those on placebo but for those on natural conjugated oestrogens the survival rate was better than placebo, especially with respect to deaths from ischaemic heart disease. Paradoxically, administration of the synthetic oestrogens resulted in a lowering of serum cholesterol whereas the natural oestrogens, which appeared to improve survival, had no effect on serum cholesterol.

The latter were the only two trials to have suggested beneficial results of oestrogens in men. Subsequent larger and, in some cases, better-designed trials showed either no benefit or deleterious effects. That oestrogen might have a harmful effect was suggested by two studies published in 1967. 167 patients with cerebrovascular disease or cerebral infarction, average age 64, 70% of whom were male and 35% of whom had diabetes, were entered into a trial of premarin, 1.25 mg, or placebo[55]. In follow-up ranging from 6 months to 3 years no prophylactic effect on the occurrence of cerebrovascular disease or myocardial infarction was found. Indeed, deaths from cerebrovascular disease and myocardial infarction were much more common in the treated groups. A harmful effect of oestrogens in men was also suggested by the Veterans Administration Co-operative Urological Research Group[56] who reported that men treated with oestrogens for carcinoma of the prostate had an increased mortality from cardiovascular disease. The Coronary Drug Project was a large double-blind randomized control trial of a number of different preparations for lowering serum lipids. The subjects studied were all men aged 30–64 years who had previous myocardial infarction at least 3 months beforehand. Two doses of oestrogen were used, and it was reported early that 5 mg of conjugated equine oestrogens per day was associated with an excess of non-fatal myocardial infarction, pulmonary embolism and thrombophlebitis[57]. The lower dose of oestrogen, 2.5 mg/day, was continued for 5 years. Treatment with this dose of oestrogen resulted in no difference in deaths from all causes or deaths from cardiovascular disease, myocardial infarction or coronary heart disease. Deaths from pulmonary embolism were more frequent in the treatment group, although the difference was not significant, and there also was a trend to higher cancer mortality in the treatment groups[58].

At best, oestrogen therapy appears to have no effect in the prevention of further progression of atherosclerotic vascular disease in men despite beneficial effects on serum cholesterol. Since the effect on vascular disease is minimal, whereas the effect on serum cholesterol is significant, oestrogen therapy may be promoting vascular disease by some other means. The increased incidence of venous thromboembolism raises the possibility that oestrogen therapy may have some effect on blood-clotting mechanisms. There have been no studies of oestrogens in the primary prevention of myocardial infarction in men. In view of the disappointing results of the secondary prevention studies, it is unlikely that such investigations will be carried out.

CONCLUSIONS

It is probably naive to suggest that conclusions can be drawn on the relationship of sex hormones to cardiovascular disease. The type of hormone, its chemical composition, dose and duration of use are all important variables. Combinations of hormones have effects which may not reflect the actions of the individual components. The hormonal status of the recipient, whether male or female, and if female, whether pre- or postmenopausal, is also important. Thus, it may be that in certain people a sex hormone of particular chemical composition, in a particular dose and for a specified time, will have deleterious effects on the cardiovascular system. At present it is not possible to make such definite statements and the only conclusions that can be drawn are broad generalizations.

The risk of myocardial infarction is increased in women who use oral contraceptives. The risk of stroke and subarachnoid haemorrhage is probably also increased but the evidence is less conclusive. The risk appears to be greater in older women and in smokers, and continues for several years after discontinuation of the preparations. The risk of myocardial infarction is related to the dose of both the oestrogen and progestogen components of the pill. The pathological changes in the artery are not clear, but it is likely that atherosclerosis occurs although thrombosis is probably also involved.

Whether postmenopausal oestrogen therapy is beneficial, harmful or of no effect on the cardiovascular system is not clear. The type and dose of the preparation and the hormonal status of the recipient are probably all important variables. The results in men were also variable although it seems clear that high doses of oestrogen have harmful effects.

Overall there is little evidence in favour of oestrogens having a preventative effect in cardiovascular disease and, at least in oral contraceptives, they increase the risk of myocardial infarction. This is difficult to reconcile with the apparent protective effects of the female sex against atherosclerosis at least in the younger age groups.

References

1. Stadel, B. V. (1981). Oral contraceptives and cardiovascular disease. *N. Engl. J. Med.*, **305**, 612 and 672
2. Vessey, M. P. (1980). Female hormones and vascular disease – an epidemiological overview. *Br. J. Fam. Plan.*, **6**, 1
3. Radford, D. J. and Oliver, M. F. (1973). Oral contraceptives and myocardial infarction. *Br. Med. J.*, **3**, 428
4. Mann, J. I., Vessey, M. P., Thorogood, M. and Doll, R. (1975). Myocardial infarction in young women with special reference to oral contraceptive practice. *Br. Med J.*, **2**, 241
5. Mann, J. I., Thorogood, M., Waters, W. E. and Powell, C. (1975). Oral contraceptives and myocardial infarction in young women: a further report. *Br. Med J.*, **3**, 631
6. Mann, J. I. and Inman, W. H. W. (1975). Oral contraceptives and death from myocardial infarction. *Br. Med J.*, **2**, 245
7. Mann, J. I., Inman, W. H. W. and Thorogood, M. (1976). Oral contraceptive use in older women and fatal myocardial infarction. *Br. Med. J.*, **2**, 445
8. Shapiro, S., Shone, D., Rosenberg, L., Kaufman, D. W., Stolley, P. D. and Miettinen, O. S. (1979). Oral contraceptive use in relation to myocardial infarction. *Lancet*, **1**, 743
9. Jick, H., Dinan, B. and Rothman, K. J. (1978). Oral contraceptives and nonfatal myocardial infarction. *J. Am. Med. Assoc.*, **239**, 1403
10. Petitti, D. B., Wingerd, J., Pellegrin, F. and Ramcharan, S. (1979). Risk of vascular disease in women. *J. Am. Med. Assoc.*, **242**, 1150
11. Royal College of General Practitioners' Oral Contraception Study (1981). Further analyses of mortality in oral contraceptive users. *Lancet*, **1**, 541
12. Krueger, D. E., Ellenberg, S. S., Bloom, S. *et al.* (1980). Fatal myocardial infarction and the role of oral contraceptives. *Am. J. Epidemiol.*, **111**, 655
13. Royal College of General Practitioners (1977). Mortality among oral contraceptive users. *Lancet*, **2**, 727
14. Vessey, M., Doll, R., Peto, R., Johnson, B. and Wiggins, P. (1976). A long term follow-up study of women using different methods of contraception – an interim report. *J. Biosoc. Sci.*, **8**, 373
15. Vessey, M. P., McPherson, K. and Johnson, B. (1977). Mortality among women participating in the Oxford/Family Planning Association contraceptive study. *Lancet*, **2**, 731

16. Vessey, M. P., McPherson, K. and Yeates, D. (1981). Mortality in oral contraceptive users. *Lancet*, **1**, 549

17. Slone, D., Shapiro, S., Kaufman, D. W., Rosenberg, L., Miettinen, O. S. and Stolley, P. D. (1981). Risk of myocardial infarction in relation to current and discontinued use of oral contraceptives. *N. Engl. J. Med.*, **305**, 420

18. Meade, T. W., Greenberg, G. and Thompson, S. G. (1980). Progestogens and cardiovascular reactions associated with oral contraceptives and a comparison of the safety of 50- and 30-μg oestrogen preparations. *Br. Med. J.*, **280**, 1157

19. Collaborative Group for the study of stroke in young women (1973). Oral contraceptives and increased risk of cerebral ischaemia or thrombosis. *N. Engl. J. Med.*, **288**, 871

20. Irey, N. N. and Norris, H. J. (1973). Intimal vascular lesions associated with female reproductive steroids. *Arch. Pathol.*, **96**, 227

21. Irey, N. N., Manion, W. C. and Taylor, H. B. (1970). Vascular lesions in women taking oral contraceptives. *Arch. Pathol.*, **89**, 1

22. Gammel, E. B. (1976). Intimal thickening in arteries of rats treated with synthetic sex hormones. *Br. J. Exp. Pathol.*, **57**, 248

23. Spain, D. M. (1978). Concerning the pathology of acute coronary heart disease in young women. In Oliver, M. F. (ed.) *Coronary Heart Disease in Young Women*, pp. 61–70. (Edinburgh: Churchill Livingstone)

24. Weir, R. J., Briggs, E., Mack, A., Naiswith, L., Taylor, L. and Wilson, E. (1974). Blood pressure in women taking oral contraceptives. *Br. Med. J.*, **1**, 533

25. Stern, M. P., Brown, B. W., Haskell, W. L., Farquhar, J. W., Wehrle, C. L. and Wood, P. D. S. (1976). Cardiovascular risk and use of estrogens or estrogen-progestagen combinations. *J. Am. Med. Assoc.*, **235**, 811

26. Ostrander, L. D. Jr, Lamphiear, D. E., Block, W. D., Williams, G. W. and Carmen, W. J. (1980). Oral contraceptives and physiological variables. *J. Am. Med. Assoc.*, **244**, 677

27. Bengtsson, C. (1977). Arterial hypertension as a risk factor for ischemic heart disease in women – results from a retrospective and from a prospective study. *Acta Med. Scand.*, suppl. **602**, 44

28. Kannel, W. B., Schwartz, M. J. and McNamara, P. M. (1969). Blood pressure and risk of coronary disease. The Framingham study. *Dis. Chest*, **56**, 43

29. Kannel, W. B., Wolf, P. A., Verter, J. and McNamara, P. M. (1970). Epidemiologic assessment of the role of blood pressure in stroke. The Framingham study. *J. Am. Med. Assoc.*, **214**, 301

30. Engel, H. J., Hundeshagen, H. and Lichtlen, P. (1977). Transmural myocardial infarction in young women taking oral contraceptives. Evidence of reduced regional coronary flow in spite of normal coronary arteries. *Br. Heart J.*, **39**, 477

31. Bolton, G. H., Hampton, J. R. and Mitchell, J. R. A. (1968). Effect of oral contraceptive agents on platelets and plasma phospholipids. *Lancet*, **1**, 1336

32. Poller, L., Priest, C. M. and Thompson, J. M. (1969). Platelet aggregation during oral contraception. *Br. Med. J.*, **4**, 273

33. Elkeles, R. S., Hampton, J. R. and Mitchell, J. R. A. (1968). Effects of oestrogen on human platelet behaviour. *Lancet*, **2**, 315

34. Poller, L. (1976). Oral contraception and blood clotting. In Gillingham, F. J., Maudsley, C. and Williams, A. E. (eds.) *Stroke*, pp. 315–46. (Edinburgh: Churchill Livingstone)

35. Meade, T. W., Chakrabarti, R., Haines, A. P., Howarth, D. J., North, W. R. S. and Stirling, Y. (1977). Haemostatic, lipid and blood-pressure profiles of women on oral contraceptives containing 50 mg or 30 mg oestrogen. *Lancet*, **2**, 948

36. Carvalho, A. C. A., Vaillancourt, R. A., Cabral, R. B., Lees, R. S. and Colman, R. W. (1977). Coagulation abnormalities in women taking oral contraceptives. *J. Am. Med. Assoc.*, **237**, 875

37. Wessler, S. (1980). Thrombosis and sex hormones: a perplexing liaison. *J. Lab. Clin. Med.*, **96**, 759

38. Rosenberg, L., Armstrong, B. and Jick, H. (1976). Myocardial infarction and estrogen therapy in postmenopausal women. *N. Engl. J. Med.*, **294**, 1256

39. Pfeffer, R. I. and Van der Neort, S. (1976). Estrogen use and stroke risk in postmenopausal women. *Am. J. Epidemiol.*, **103**, 445

40. Pfeffer, R. I., Whipple, G. H., Kurosaki, T. T. and Chapman, J. M. (1978). Coronary risk

and estrogen use in postmenopausal women. *Am. J. Epidemiol.*, **107**, 479

41. Rosenberg, L., Slone, D., Shapiro, S., Kaufman, D., Stolley, P. D. and Miettinen, O. S. (1980). Noncontraceptive estrogens and myocardial infarction in young women. *J. Am. Med. Assoc.*, **244**, 339

42. Bain, C., Willett, W., Hennekens, C. H., Rosner, B., Belanger, C. and Speizer, F. E. (1981). Use of postmenopausal hormones and risk of myocardial infarction *Circulation*, **64**, 42

43. Adam, S., Williams, V. and Vessey, M. P. (1981). Cardiovascular disease and hormone replacement treatment: a pilot case control study. *Br. Med. J.*, **282**, 1277

44. Gordon, T., Kannel, W. B., Hjortland, M. C. and McNamara, P. M. (1978). Menopause and coronary heart disease. The Framingham study. *Ann. Intern. Med.*, **89**, 157

45. Jick, H., Dinan, B. and Rothman, K. J. (1978). Noncontraceptive estrogens and nonfatal myocardial infarction. *J. Am. Med. Assoc.*, **239**, 1407

46. Jick, H., Dinan, B. and Rothman, K. J. (1978). Myocardial infarction and other vascular diseases in young women. *J. Am. Med. Assoc.*, **240**, 2548

47. Ross, R. K., Paganni-Hill, A., Mack, T. M., Arthur, M. and Henderson, B. E. (1981). Menopausal oestrogen therapy and protection from death from ischaemic heart disease. *Lancet*, **1**, 858

48. Wallace, R. B., Hoover, J., Sandler, D., Rifkind, B. M. and Tyroler, H. A. (1977). Altered plasma-lipids associated with oral contraceptive or oestrogen consumption. *Lancet*, **2**, 11

49. Barrett-Connor, E., Brown, V., Turner, J., Austin, M. and Criqui, M. H. (1979). Heart disease risk factors and hormone use in postmenopausal women. *J. Am. Med. Assoc.*, **24**, 2167

50. Hammond, C. B., Jelovsek, F. R., Lee, K. L., Creasman, W. T. and Parker, R. T. (1979). Effects of long-term estrogen replacement therapy. *Am. J. Obstet. Gynecol.*, **133**, 525

51. Lindquist, O. and Bengtsson, C. (1980). Serum lipids, arterial blood pressure and body weight in relation to the menopause: results from a population study of women in Goteborg, Sweden. *Scand. J. Clin. Invest.*, **40**, 629

52. Oliver, M. F. and Boyd, G. S. (1961). Influence of reduction of serum lipids on prognosis of coronary heart-disease. *Lancet*, **2**, 499

53. Stamler, J., Pick, R., Katz, L. N. *et al.* (1965). Effectiveness of estrogen for therapy of myocardial infarction in middle aged men. *J. Am. Med. Assoc.*, **183**, 632

54. Marmorstom, J., Moore, F. J., Hopkins, C. E., Kuzma, O. T. and Weiner, J. (1962). Clinical studies of long-term estrogen therapy in men with myocardial infarction. *Proc. Soc. Exp. Biol.*, **110**, 400

55. McDowell, F., Louis, S. and McDevitt, E. (1967). A clinical trial of premarin in cerebrovascular disease. *J. Chron. Dis.*, **20**, 679

56. Veterans Administration Co-operative Urological Research Group (1967). Treatment and survival of patients with cancer of the prostate. *Surg. Gynecol. Obstet.*, **124**, 1011

57. Coronary Drug Project Research Group (1970). The Coronary Drug Project. Initial findings leading to modifications of its research protocol. *J. Am. Med. Assoc.*, **214**, 1303

58. Coronary Drug Project Research Group (1973). The Coronary Drug Project. Findings leading to discontinuation of the 2.5 mg/day estrogen group. *J. Am. Med. Assoc.*, **226**, 652

11
Sex hormones, lipid and carbohydrate metabolism

LIPIDS AND LIPOPROTEINS IN MALES AND FEMALES

The marked difference in incidence of atherosclerosis in males and females, at least in developed countries, has prompted a search for differences in risk factors between the two sexes. Most attention has been paid to plasma lipids and lipoproteins and many epidemiological studies have reported differences in total and individual lipoprotein cholesterol and triglyceride in males and females.

One of the largest and most recent epidemiological studies of plasma lipids is that of the Lipid Research Clinics (LRC) Program of the National Heart, Lung and Blood Institute of the United States[1]. In this study, 12 LRCs and five support facilities were set up in the United States and Canada. The objectives of the LRCs were to acquire data on the prevalence of different types of hyperlipoproteinaemia, to collect data on the prevalence of atherosclerosis, and to conduct a trial of the effect of reduction of plasma lipids on coronary heart disease. In the study of the prevalence of hyperlipidaemia in North America the blood samples were taken after a 12 h fast and lipids were measured by standard techniques. The results of the studies on 24 425 males and 18 108 females not taking sex hormones are shown in Figure 11.1. In the younger children, plasma cholesterol is slightly higher in females than males. However, the curves cross at age 20 and from then until age 50 cholesterol is higher in males. The curves cross again at age 50 and from then cholesterol is higher in females. The pattern for plasma triglyceride is similar except that the first crossing of the curves is at age 15 and the second at age 70. The pattern of plasma lipids is thus comparable to the incidence of coronary heart disease in males and females. Similar age and sex relationships of plasma lipids have been found in smaller studies in Stockholm[2], Seattle[3] and London[4]. The higher levels of plasma cholesterol and triglyceride in childhood in females have also been found in a Danish study[5]. Kinetic studies have shown that the lower triglyceride levels in females are due to more efficient removal of the lipid from the circulation[6,7].

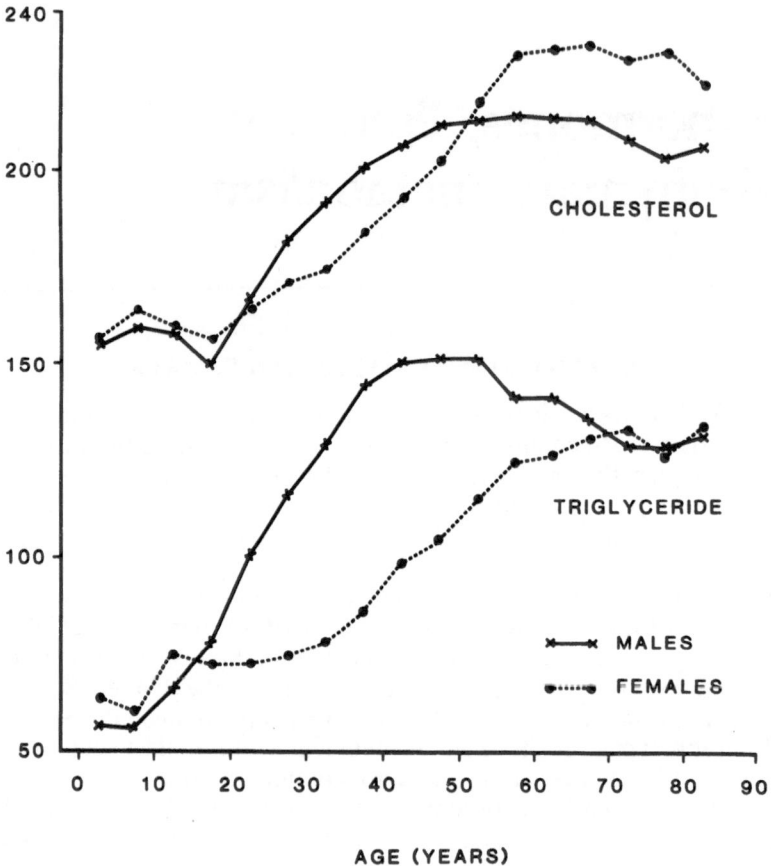

Figure 11.1   Plasma cholesterol and triglyceride levels in relation to age and sex[1]

There have been fewer studies of sex differences in lipoprotein concentrations. In Uppsala, Sweden[8], over a narrower age range than the LRC study, the general pattern of serum cholesterol and triglyceride was the same. The major part of serum cholesterol was in LDL (Figure 11.2) which showed a similar age and sex pattern to total cholesterol. HDL cholesterol was higher in females at all ages while VLDL cholesterol was higher in males up to age 60. The major part of serum triglyceride was in VLDL (Figure 11.3) which paralleled the age and sex changes of total trigylceride. There was little difference in LDL and HDL triglyceride in males and females. Somewhat similar results were found in a London study which used analytical ultracentrifugation for analysis of lipoproteins[9].

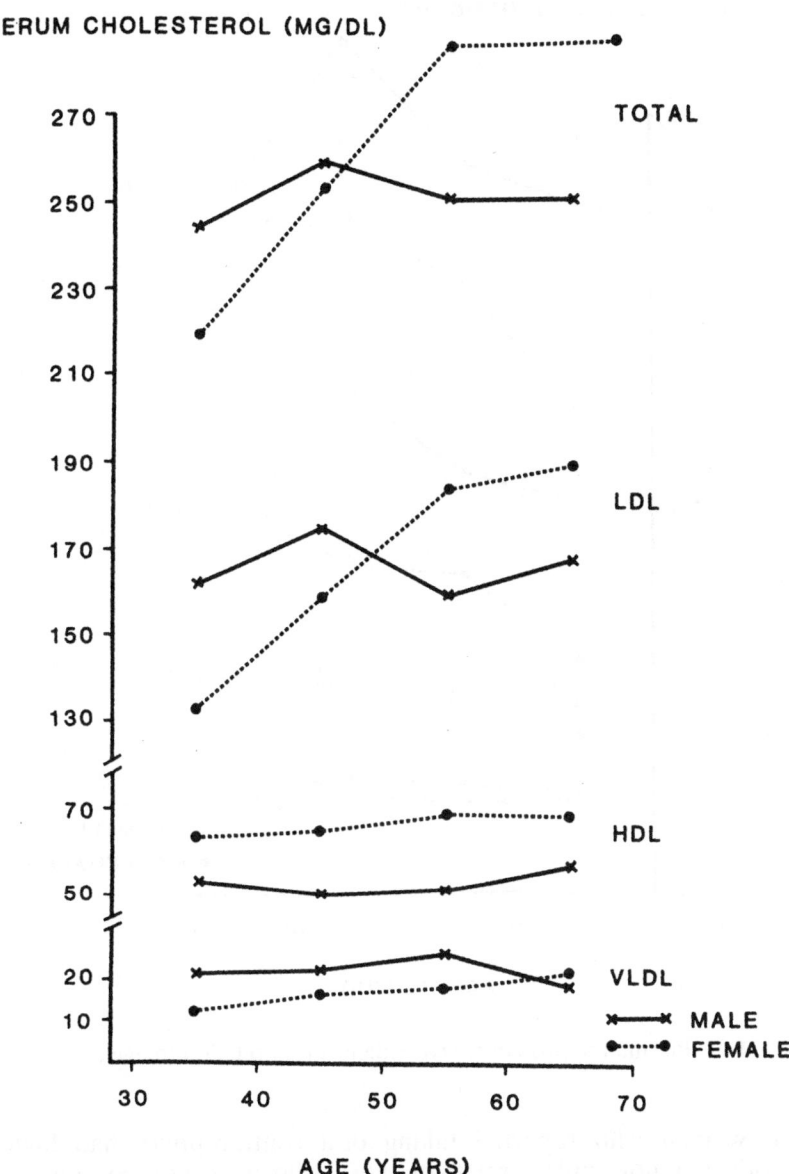

Figure 11.2 Plasma lipoprotein cholesterol levels in relation to age and sex[8]

SEX HORMONES IN LIPID METABOLISM

A large number of studies have reported abnormalities in plasma lipid
concentrations in women taking oral contraceptives. Recently some large
population studies have reported their results. In the Stanford three
community study[10], a cross-sectional study of a random sample of 986

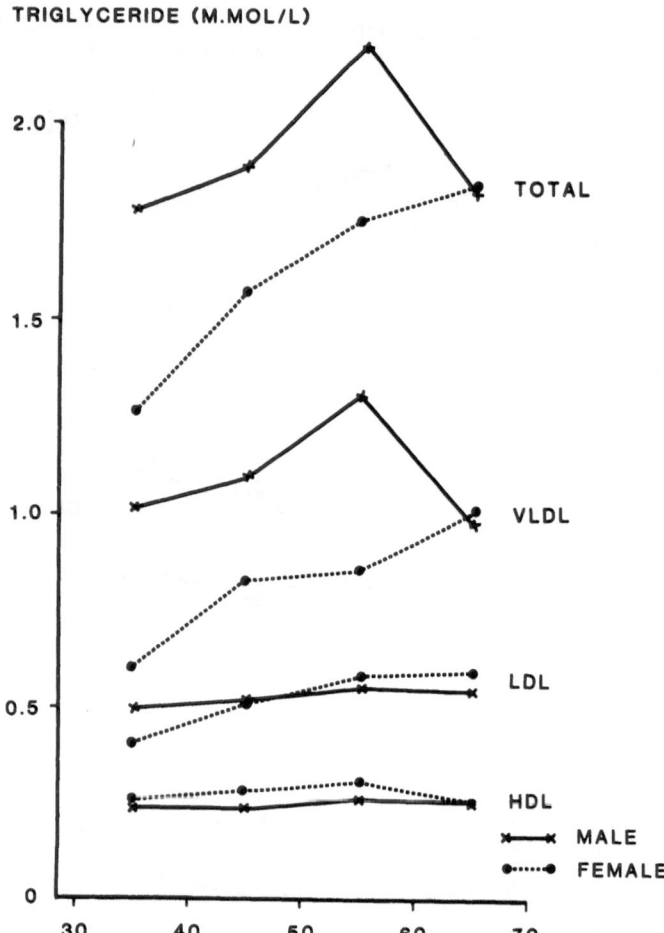

Figure 11.3   Plasma lipoprotein triglyceride levels in relation to age and sex[8]

women, women who reported taking oral contraceptives had higher triglyceride but not cholesterol than those who were not. Systolic and disastolic blood pressure were also increased in those taking oral contraceptives. Subjects who were taking oestrogen alone had similar but lesser increases in serum triglycerides. In the Lipid Research Clinic Program[11] 18 461 white non-pregnant women were studied. 50% of white females aged 20–24 were taking oral contraceptives. Triglyceride was elevated by an average of 48% (33–40 mg/dl) and cholesterol by an average of 5% (12–15 mg/dl) in those taking the hormone preparations compared to non-users (Figure 11.4). Hypertriglyceridaemia was 5 times as common and hypercholesterolaemia 3 times as common in users than non-users. 37% of

PLASMA LIPIDS (MG/DL)

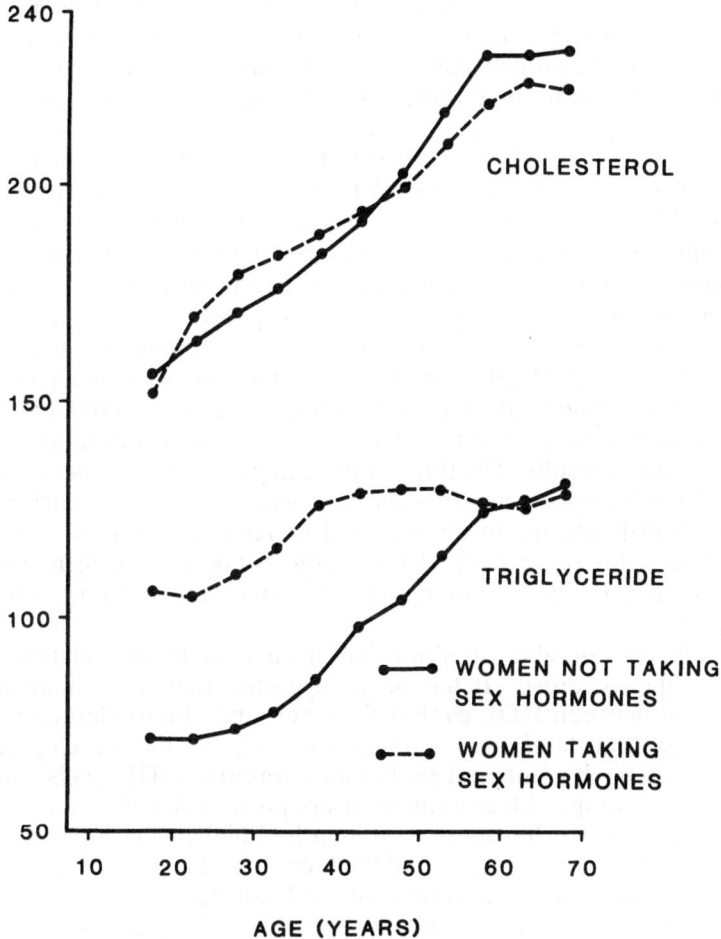

Figure 11.4   Effect of oral contraceptives on plasma cholesterol and triglyceride[11]

older women, aged 50–54 years, were hormone users but there was a much smaller change (5% – 5–10 mg/dl) in triglyceride and a slight fall (5–6% – 10–12 mg/dl) in cholesterol in these women. This may be because these women were taking oestrogen alone as postmenopausal hormone replacement therapy. It was not possible in either of the two community studies to identify the composition of the drugs which were taken. The LRC Program analysed in more detail a 15% random sample of the study population[12]. In these 2606 women, users of oral contraceptives had significantly higher total cholesterol (2–16 mg/dl) and total triglyceride (30–60 mg/dl) levels over those of non-users. Oral contraceptive users had higher VLDL cholesterol and younger users had higher LDL cholesterol levels. There was no effect on HDL cholesterol. When the oestrogen content of the hormone preparations was considered, plasma total cholesterol, total triglyceride and VLDL cholesterol levels rose with increasing oestrogen content but there was no relation between LDL cholesterol and oestrogen content. HDL cholesterol was only elevated above levels in non-users in those taking the highest dose of oestrogen. In contrast, older women taking oestrogen alone had lower cholesterol and slightly lower triglyceride levels than non-users. Oestrogen users had lower LDL cholesterol, slightly lower VLDL cholesterol and higher HDL cholesterol levels than non-users. Thus, except for HDL, the effects of oral contraceptives are different to those of oestrogen alone. This suggests that the effects of the combined preparations may be due to the progestogen components. However, differences in the responses of younger and older women to oestrogen must also be considered. A community study of 190 white women aged 21–39[13] found that triglyceride was 19 mg/dl (26%) higher in oral contraceptive users but total cholesterol and HDL cholesterol were not significantly different. Drugs of different composition showed slightly different results. The three American population studies thus agree that oral contraceptive use is associated with raised plasma triglyceride levels with little change in plasma total or HDL cholesterol. The raised triglyceride is due to a rise in VLDL. Subjects taking oestrogen alone had lesser changes in lipids and lipoproteins than those taking combined preparations.

Recently considerable attention has been paid to the relationship of HDL to atherosclerosis. It has been suggested that there is an inverse relationship between HDL cholesterol levels and atherosclerotic vascular disease and that HDL has a protective role in the development of atherosclerosis[14]. A number of studies have reported HDL levels in women on hormone therapy. Measurement of apoprotein A–I the major protein component of HDL showed that women had higher levels than men but women who were on oestrogen had the highest A–I levels, the next highest being those who were on combined oral contraceptive preparations.[15] Oestrogen therapy increased apoprotein A–I levels by about 24%. In the Walnut Creek Contraceptive Drug Study[16], a cross-sectional study of 4978 women aged 21–62, HDL cholesterol increased by about 2 mg/dl per decade. Increase in weight and smoking were associated with a fall in HDL and alcohol with a rise. After allowing for these variables, HDL levels were positively correlated with oestrogen dose and inversely correlated with progestogen dose. Combined oral contraceptive preparations had intermediate effects which varied with the composition of the preparation. On the other hand, another community study[17] found that although HDL was higher in women than in men, and smoking reduced HDL in both women and men, oral contraceptive users had reduced HDL levels. A detailed study of lipoprotein changes in 18 women aged 20–39 years from the Walnut Creek study has shown that oral contraceptive use is associated with a rise in HDL which was due to an increase in the denser HDL$_3$ subfraction[18]. The different results in these studies may be explained by the effects of differing oral contraceptive composition on lipids and lipoproteins[19]. The route and type of oestrogen administration also influences the effect on lipids and lipoproteins[20].

High doses of oestrogens administered to men for the treatment of prostatic carcinoma resulted in a slight decrease in plasma total cholesterol and a 50–60% increase in HDL cholesterol[21,22]. Triglyceride increased about 40%. Orchidectomy resulted in only slight changes in lipids and lipoproteins.

Studies of the relation of endogenous sex hormone levels to lipids and lipoproteins have produced conflicting results. A positive correlation between serum testosterone and HDL cholesterol was found in a group of 26 men[23], in 150 men in a population study[24], in a group of azoospermic, oligospermic and normal young men[25] and in 247 middle-aged men[26]. However no correlation between testosterone and HDL was found in 79 male diabetics[27]. In the diabetics, oestradiol correlated with HDL, but no correlation of HDL with either oestradiol or oestrone was found in two other studies[23,24]. Testosterone was negatively correlated with triglyceride and VLDL cholesterol in four studies[24-27] and positively correlated with total cholesterol in one[23]. Oestradiol correlated negatively with LDL and LDL cholesterol in the diabetics. Further studies are required to clarify the relation of endogenous sex hormone secretion with lipids and lipoproteins. The positive association of testosterone and HDL appears inconsistent with the association of coronary heart disease with both HDL and the male sex.

Effect of hormone preparation, dose and potency

The possibility that different oestrogens and progestogens have different effects on lipid and lipoprotein metabolism has been the subject of a number of studies (Table 11.1). A British study[28] of 1628 women taking six different types of oral contraceptives found elevation of serum cholesterol only with pills containing $75 \mu g$ or more oestrogen and an oestrane progestogen. Serum cholesterol tended to be lower if the preparation contained a gonane progestogen. Triglyceride elevations were oestrogen-dose related. As a raised cholesterol was only found with the highest oestrogen dose, this is further evidence that VLDL is the lipoprotein predominantly affected by oestrogens. Pregnane progestogens potentiated the effect of oestrogens on triglyceride levels while gonane progestogens antagonized them. Oral contraceptives containing $75 \mu g$ of oestrogen are no longer available. With a modern low-dose ($30 \mu g$) oestrogen oral contraceptive, there was a small (7%) but significant rise in plasma total cholesterol but no change in triglycerides or LDL, VLDL, or HDL cholesterol[29]. In a study of telephone company employees[30] total VLDL and HDL triglyceride increased with increasing oestrogen potency but LDL triglyceride was not related to oestrogen potency. LDL cholesterol was elevated in women taking oral contraceptives but was lower than controls in those taking postmenopausal oestrogen therapy. HDL cholesterol was highest with high oestrogen potency. In addition, lipoprotein composition was altered by sex hormone treatment. It was concluded that the response of lipids and lipoproteins to sex hormones

Table 11.1 Synthetic oestrogens and progestogens used in oral contraceptives[28]

Oestrogens
Two synthetic oestrogens are used in oral contraceptives – ethinyl oestradiol and mestranol, the 3-methyl ether of ethinyl oestradiol. Mestranol is inactive until converted to ethinyl oestradiol by the liver.

Progestogens
Synthetic progestogens are:

Pregnanes (Megestrol, chlormadinone, and medroxyprogesterone acetate); no oral contraceptive containing a pregnane is now available

Oestranes (Norethisterone, norethisterone acetate, lynoestranol, ethynodiol diacetate and norethynodrel); the oestrane progestogens (19-nortestosterone progestogens) are all metabolized to norethisterone before becoming active

Gonane (Nogestrel); the gonane is an active progestogen without metabolic transformation

---

depends on the composition and the potency of the preparations used.

The effect of different progestogens on lipoproteins has been studied in three groups of postmenopausal women[31]. The groups were matched for lipid levels and all other factors which might have influenced the results. All were started on oestradiol for 1 month. The effect of this was to increase total cholesterol and LDL cholesterol and to increase HDL cholesterol in some patients. After this the subjects were assigned to three different progestogens, norethindrone acetate (an oestrane) 10 mg daily, medroxyprogesterone (a pregnane) 10 mg daily, and norgestrel (a gonane) 0.5 mg daily. With combined treatment total cholesterol decreased in all groups by 10–18% of baseline values, the greatest decrease occurring in women who had high initial concentrations. HDL cholesterol concentrations decreased by 20% from baseline after only 1 month of combined treatment with norethindrone and with norgestrel but no significant change occurred with medroxyprogesterone. The magnitude of the HDL cholesterol changes was not related to the initial value. There was a slight though statistically insignificant decrease in LDL cholesterol during the period. Triglyceride decreased significantly only with norgestrel. These results show that the effects of different components of hormone preparations have to be considered and that progestogens in general have effects which are opposite to those of oestrogens.

Androgens have similar effects to progestogens on lipid metabolism lowering triglyceride levels[32,33] and increasing the activities of the enzymes hepatic lipase and phospholipase A[34]. The results of human[32,35] and animal[36] studies show that androgens lower VLDL triglyceride levels by increasing triglyceride removal from the circulation.

Mechanism of lipid changes

The mechanism by which oral contraceptives alter plasma lipid metabolism has been studied in a number of different ways, with considerable agreement on the results. A combination of ethinyloestradiol and medroxyprogesterone for 2 weeks caused a 47% rise in plasma triglyceride levels but a 46% fall in post-heparin lipolytic activity[37]. The latter represents the activity of the enzyme lipoprotein lipase, the major enzyme responsible for triglyceride catabolism in the circulation. Basal insulin levels were increased by 59%. Despite the defect in enzyme activity it was suggested that increased triglyceride synthesis was the mechanism by which triglyceride levels were increased by oral contraceptives. Oestrogen alone had similar effects to the combined preparation. A more detailed investigation of the effect of oestrogen on triglyceride metabolism was reported by the same laboratory[38]. Normal women were given 1 μg/kg of ethinyloestradiol daily for 2 weeks. Although triglyceride rose by 76% and hepatic triglyceride lipase decreased by 68%, adipose tissue lipoprotein lipase was not significantly changed. It was concluded that the previously reported decrease in post-heparin lipolytic activity represented hepatic triglyceride lipase. There was no correlation between the change in hepatic lipase and the change in triglyceride levels, suggesting that hepatic lipase had probably little effect on triglyceride removal. It was concluded that the increase in triglyceride associated with oestrogen use was due to increased production of the lipid.

A study of plasma triglyceride turnover showed that different preparations of oral contraceptives resulted in raised serum triglyceride levels, increased triglyceride production and increased triglyceride removal. It was concluded that the raised triglyceride levels were due to increased influx and this was partly compensated by increased triglyceride efflux[39]. Another study of triglyceride turnover using a different technique found that combined contraceptives or oestrogen alone caused a rise in triglyceride and triglyceride turnover but progestogen, on the other hand, caused a decrease in triglyceride levels[40]. A Swedish study looked at the effects of oestrogen and progestogen on lipid transport[41]. A combined preparation containing the oestrogen mestranol 0.1 mg caused a 200% rise in triglyceride, a 10–20% rise in cholesterol, a rise in VLDL levels and a fall in post-heparin lipolytic activity. The intravenous fat tolerance test was unchanged, suggesting that the increase in triglyceride levels was due to increased triglyceride influx into the circulation. When the combined preparation was replaced by progestogen, triglyceride and cholesterol levels fell, suggesting that it was the oestrogen which resulted in the lipid changes. The kinetic studies are thus in fairly close agreement, suggesting that oral contraceptives, and in particular the oestrogen component, cause a rise in triglyceride levels resulting from an increase in triglyceride synthesis and delivery into the circulation. There is also an increase in triglyceride removal but this is not great enough to compensate for the increased influx. The effect on cholesterol is small and may be secondary to the effect on triglyceride-rich lipoproteins. It appears that oestrogen is particularly responsible for the rise in triglyceride levels while progestogen has the opposite effect. Combined preparations have different effects depending on their composition. The mechanism of the changes in HDL has not been investigated.

An exception to oestrogen's effect in raising triglyceride and cholesterol levels occurs in type III hyperlipoproteinaemia. This rare inherited disorder of lipid metabolism is characterized by elevated triglyceride and cholesterol levels and by the presence in the circulation of 'remnant' or intermediate-density lipoprotein particles which have the characteristics of cholesterol-rich, β-migrating VLDL. Remnants are formed by the removal of triglyceride from VLDL by the enzyme lipoprotein lipase. Type III hyperlipoproteinaemia is thought to be due to a defect in the hepatic catabolism of remnants to LDL[42]. Oestrogens lower triglyceride and cholesterol levels in type III hyperlipoproteinaemia and correct the abnormal lipoprotein composition[43]. Oestrogens act by stimulating remnant catabolism[42], probably by way of increasing remnant uptake by the liver[44].

CARBOHYDRATE METABOLISM

Soon after the widespread introduction of oral contraceptives it was shown that they cause abnormalities in carbohydrate metabolism including impaired glucose tolerance and hypo- or hyperinsulinism[45-47]. As with lipid metabolism the effects of oral contraceptives on blood glucose and serum insulin levels vary with the composition of the pill. In a large study of the effects of six different oral contraceptive combinations[28] fasting plasma glucose was lower with all six than in age-matched controls and oral glucose tolerance impaired with all except the preparation containing a pregnane progestogen. The greatest impairment of oral glucose tolerance occurred with preparations with the highest oestrogen content. The fasting and post-glucose insulin levels were elevated with all preparations except those containing pregnane progestogens. With the high oestrogen dose the early insulin response to glucose was impaired. The highest insulin responses were found with preparations containing gonane progestogens. When related to plasma glucose levels, oral contraceptives with a high oestrogen content had a reduced insulin response while oestrane or gonane progestogens had elevated insulin responses. With the pregnane progestogen the response was the same as the control. The authors suggest that since oestrogens alone do not alter glucose tolerance, the diabetogenic effect may be due to the progestogen. In most cases the impaired glucose tolerance is associated with insulin resistance. The effect of progestogen on insulin secretion was confirmed in the rat in which progesterone treatment resulted in an increased insulin response to glucose or arginine[48]. In contrast, pancreatic glucagon responses to arginine were unchanged. Oral contraceptives containing very low doses of an oestrane progestogen, either alone or in combination with 50 μg of ethinyl oestradiol, have no effect on glucose or insulin responses to oral glucose tolerance tests[49]. Lower fasting glucose levels were also found in a large population study of users of postmenopausal oestrogens[50]. A study of 270 women aged 30–59 years selected at random from the Tecumseh study showed that the 20 who were current users of oral contraceptives had higher glucose and insulin responses to glucose challenge than non-users or former users[51]. It appears, therefore, that oral contraceptives cause insulin resistance resulting in hyperglycaemia and compensatory elevations in insulin levels. The exact responses depend on the composition of the preparations, the progestogen being the most important component.

CONCLUSIONS

Plasma cholesterol and triglyceride levels are higher in males between the ages of about 15 and 60 years. These are due to changes in LDL and VLDL respectively. HDL cholesterol is higher in adult females. Lipids and lipoproteins in males and females reflect the incidence of atherosclerosis in the sexes.

Oral contraceptives increase triglyceride and VLDL levels and have little effects on LDL. However the effect varies with the composition of the preparations and with the dose and potency of the hormones. In general, oestrogens and progestogens have opposite effects on lipid metabolism. Oestrogens increase triglyceride synthesis and have a smaller effect on triglyceride removal. However, oestrogens also increase the uptake of lipoprotein remnants by the liver, reducing triglyceride and cholesterol levels in type III hyperlipidaemia.

While the sex differences in lipids and lipoproteins reflect the sex differences in atherosclerosis, the effect of exogenous sex hormones on lipid metabolism are less easy to relate to cardiovascular disease. Thus, the relation of oral contraceptives to cardiovascular disease is not clearly related to the effect of these drugs on lipid metabolism. The changes in carbohydrate metabolism, which occur with oral contraceptive use, with hyperglycaemia and hyperinsulinaemia, are similar to those associated with atherosclerosis in other circumstances.

References

1. Lipid Research Clinics Program Epidemiology Committee (1979). Plasma lipid distributions in selected North American populations: the lipid research clinics program prevalence study. *Circulation*, **60**, 427
2. Carlson, L. A. and Lindsted, S. (1969). The Stockholm Prospective Study. I. The initial values for plasma lipids. *Acta Med. Scand.*, **185**, (suppl. 493), 1
3. Goldstein, J. L., Hazzard, W. R., Schrott, H. G., Bierman, E. L. and Motulsky, A. G. (1973). Hyperlipidemia in coronary heart disease. Lipid levels in 500 survivors of myocardial infarction. *J. Clin. Invest.*, **52**, 1533
4. Lewis, B., Chait, A., Wooton, I. D. P. *et al.* (1974). Frequency of risk factors for ischaemic heart-disease in a healthy British population. *Lancet*, **1**, 141
5. Dyerberg, J. and Hjorne, N. (1973). Plasma lipid and lipoprotein levels in childhood and adolescence. *Scand. J. Clin. Lab. Invest.*, **31**, 473
6. Nikkila, E. A. and Kekki, M. (1971). Polymorphism of plasma triglyceride kinetics in normal human adult subjects. *Acta Med. Scand.*, **190**, 49
7. Olefsky, J., Farquhar, J. W. and Reaven, G. M. (1974). Sex difference in kinetics of triglyceride metabolism in normal and hypertriglyceridaemic human subjects. *Eur. J. Clin. Invest.*, **4**, 121

8. Carlson, L. A. and Ericsson, M. (1975). Quantitative and qualitative serum lipoprotein analysis. Part 1. Studies in healthy men and women. *Atherosclerosis*, **21**, 417
9. Slack, J., Noble, N., Meade, T. W. and North, W. R. S. (1977). Lipid and lipoprotein concentrations in 1604 men and women in working populations in north-west London. *Br. Med. J.*, **2**, 353
10. Stern, M. P., Brown, B. W., Jr, Haskell, W. L., Farquhar, J. W., Wehrle, C. L. and Wood, P. D. S. (1976). Cardiovascular risk and use of oestrogens or oestrogen-progestogen combinations. *J. Am. Med. Assoc.*, **235**, 811
11. Wallace, R. B., Hoover, J., Sandler, D., Rifkind, B. M. and Tyroler, H. A. (1977). Altered plasma lipids associated with oral contraceptive or oestrogen consumption. *Lancet*, **2**, 11
12. Wallace, R. B., Hoover, J., Barrett-Connor, E. *et al.* (1979). Altered plasma lipid and lipoprotein levels associated with oral contraceptive and oestrogen use. *Lancet*. **2**, 111
13. Hennekens, C. H., Evans, D. A., Castelli, W. P., Taylor, J. O., Rosner, B. and Kass, E. H. (1979). Oral contraceptive use and fasting triglyceride, plasma cholesterol and HDL cholesterol. *Circulation*, **60**, 486
14. Miller, G. J. and Miller, N. E. (1975). Plasma-high density-lipoprotein concentration and development of ischaemic heart-disease. *Lancet*, **1**, 16
15. Albers, J. J., Wahl, P. W., Cabana, V. G., Hazzard, W. R. and Hoover, J. J. (1976). Quantitation of apolipoprotein A–I of human plasma high density lipoprotein. *Metabolism*, **25**, 633
16. Bradley, D. D., Wingerd, J., Petitti, D. A., Kraus, R. M. and Raucharan, S. (1978). Serum high-density-lipoprotein cholesterol in women using oral contraceptives, estrogens and progestogens. *N. Engl. J. Med.*, **299**, 17
17. Arntzenius, A. C., van Gent, C. M., van der Voort, H., Stegerhoek, C. I. and Styblo, K. (1978). Reduced high-density lipoprotein in women aged 40–41 using oral contraceptives. *Lancet*, **1**, 1221
18. Krauss, R. M., Lindgren, F. T., Silvers, A., Jutagir, R. and Bradley, D. D. (1977) Changes in serum high density lipoproteins in women on oral contraceptive drugs. *Clin. Chim. Acta*, **80**, 465
19. Larsson-Cohn, U., Wallentin, L. and Zador, G. (1979). Plasma lipids and high density lipoproteins during oral contraception with different combinations of ethinyl estradiol and levonorgestrel. *Horm. Metab. Res.*, **11**, 437
20. Buckman, M. T., Johnson, J., Ellis, H., Srivastava, L. and Peake, G. T. (1980). Differential lipemic and proteinemic response to oral ethinyl estradiol and parenteral estradiol cypionate. *Metabolism*, **29**, 803
21. Wallentin, L. and Varenhorst, E. (1978). Changes of plasma lipid metabolism in males during estrogen treatment for prostatic carcinoma. *J. Clin. Endocrinol. Metab.*, **47**, 596
22. Wallentin, L. and Varenhorst, E. (1981). Plasma lipoproteins during anti-androgen treatment by estrogens or orchidectomy in men with prostatic carcinoma. *Horm. Metab. Res.*, **13**, 293
23. Nordoy, A., Aakvaag, A. and Thelle, D. (1979). Sex hormones and high density lipoproteins in healthy males. *Atherosclerosis*, **34**, 431
24. Heller, R. F., Miller, N. E., Lewis, B. *et al.* (1981) Associations between sex hormones, thyroid hormones and lipoproteins. *Clin. Sci.*, **61**, 649
25. Mendozza, S. G., Osuna, A., Zerpa, A., Gartside, P. S. and Glueck, C. J. (1981). Hypertriglyceridemia and hypoalphalipoproteinemia in azoospermic and oligospermic young men: relationships of endogenous testosterone to triglyceride and high density lipoprotein cholesterol metabolism. *Metabolism*, **30**, 481
26. Gutai, J., La Porte, R., Kuller, L., Dai, W., Falvo-Gerard, L. and Cagguila, A. (1981). Plasma testosterone, high density lipoprotein cholesterol and other lipoprotein fractions. *Am. J. Cardiol.*, **48**, 897
27. Reckless, J. P. D., Betteridge, D. J., Taylor, K. G. *et al.* (1980). Serum lipoproteins and the concentrations of thyroxine and sex hormones in diabetic man. *Horm. Metab. Res.*, **12**, 629
28. Wynn, V., Adams, P. W., Godsland, I. *et al.* (1979). Comparison of effects of different combined oral contraceptive formulations on carbohydrate and lipid metabolism. *Lancet*, **1**, 1045

29. Taggart, H. and Stout, R. W. (1981). Effect of a low dose estrogen–progestogen oral contraceptive on lipids and lipoproteins. *Irish J. Med. Sci.*, **150**, 13
30. Knopp, R. H., Walden, C. E., Wahl, P. W. *et al.* (1981). Oral contraceptive and postmenopausal estrogen effects on lipoprotein triglyceride and cholesterol in an adult female population: relationship to estrogen and progestin potency. *J. Clin. Endocrinol. Metab.*, **53**, 1123
31. Hirvonen, E., Malkonen, M. and Marninen, V. (1981). Effects of different progestogens on lipoproteins during postmenopausal replacement therapy. *N. Engl. J. Med.*, **304**, 560
32. Glueck, C. J., Ford, S., Jr., Steiner, P. and Fallat, R. (1973). Triglyceride removal efficiency and lipoprotein lipases: effects of oxandrolone. *Metabolism*, **22**, 807
33. Solyom, A. (1972). Effect of androgens on serum lipids and lipoproteins. *Lipids*, **7**, 100
34. Ehnholm, C., Huttunen, J. K., Kinnunen, P. J., Miettinen, T. A. and Nikkila, E. A. (1975). Effect of oxandrolone treatment on the activity of lipoprotein lipase, hepatic lipase and phospholipase A_1 of human postheparin plasma. *N. Engl. J. Med.*, **292**, 1314
35. Kissebah, A. H., Harrigan, P., Adams, P. W. and Wynn, V. (1973). Effect of methandienone on free fatty acid and triglyceride turnover in normal females. *Horm. Metab. Res.*, **5**, 275
36. Bagdade, J. D., Livingston, R. and Yee, E. (1975). Effects of the synthetic androgen fluoxymesterone on triglyceride secretion rates in the rat. *Proc. Soc. Exp. Biol. Med.*, **149**, 452
37. Hazzard, W. R., Spiger, M. J., Bagdade, J. D. and Bierman, E. L. (1969). Studies on the mechanism of increased plasma triglyceride levels induced by oral contraceptives. *N. Engl. J. Med.*, **280**, 471
38. Applebaum, D. M., Goldberg, A. P., Pykalisto, O. J., Brunzell, J. D. and Hazzard, W. R. (1977). Effect of estrogen on postheparin lipolytic activity. Selective decline in hepatic triglyceride lipase. *J. Clin. Invest.*, **59**, 601
39. Kekki, M. and Nikkila, E. A. (1971). Plasma triglyceride turnover during use of oral contraceptives. *Metabolism*, **20**, 878
40. Kissebah, A. H., Harrigan, P. and Wynn, V. (1973). Mechanism of hypertriglyceridaemia associated with contraceptive steroids. *Horm. Metab. Res.*, **5**, 184
41. Rossner, S., Larsson-Cohn, H., Carlson, C. A. and Boherg, J. (1971). Effects of an oral contraceptive agent on plasma lipids, plasma lipoproteins, the intravenous fat tolerance and the post-heparin lipoprotein lipase-activity. *Acta Med. Scand.*, **190**, 301
42. Chait, A., Brunzell, J. D., Albers, J. J. and Hazzard, W. R. (1977). Type III hyperlipoproteinaemia ('remnant removal disease'). *Lancet*, **1**, 1176
43. Kushwaha, R. S., Hazzard, W. R., Gagne, C., Chait A. and Albers, J. J. (1977). Type III hyperlipoproteinemia: paradoxical hypolipidemic response to estrogen. *Ann. Intern. Med.*, **87**, 517
44. Floren, C-H., Kushwaha, R. S., Hazzard, W. R. and Albers, J. J. (1981). Estrogen-induced increase in uptake of cholesterol rich very low density lipoproteins in perfused rabbit liver. *Metabolism*, **30**, 367
45. Wynn, V. and Doar, J. W. H. (1969). Some effects of oral contraceptives on carbohydrate metabolism. *Lancet*, **2**, 761
46. Wynn, V. and Doar, J. W. H. (1966). Some effects of oral contraceptives on carbohydrate metabolism. *Lancet*. **2**, 715
47. Spellacy, W. N., Buhi, W. C., Spellacy, C. E., Moses, L. E. and Goldzieher, J. W. (1970). Glucose, insulin and growth hormone studies in long-term users of oral contraceptives. *Am. J. Obstet. Gynecol.*, **106**, 173
48. Ashby, J. P., Shirling, D. and Baird, J. D. (1981). Effect of progestogen on the secretion and peripheral action of insulin and glucagon in the intact rat. *J. Endocrinol.*, **88**, 49
49. Leis, D., Bottermann, P., Ermler, R. and Schlauch, W. (1980). Effects of low-dose gestagen and combination-type oral contraception on blood glucose and serum insulin levels after a glucose load. *Arch. Gynecol.*, **230**, 143
50. Barrett-Connor, E., Brown, W. V., Turner, J., Austin, M. and Criqui, M. H. (1979). Heart disease risk factors and hormone use in postmenopausal woman. *J. Am. Med. Assoc.*, **241**, 2167
51. Ostrander, L. D., Lamphiear, D. E., Block, W. D., Williams, G. W. and Carmen, W. J. (1980). Oral contraceptives and physiological variables. *J. Am. Med. Assoc.*, **244**, 677

12
The effects of sex hormones on the arterial wall

In the past 40 years there have been a number of studies of the effect of sex hormones on the arterial wall. The earlier studies looked at the effect of administering sex hormones to whole animals which were often also fed high-fat diets. Later the direct effects of sex hormones on isolated arterial tissue or cultured arterial cells were investigated. The results have not always been consistent with each other or with clinical observations, and much still remains to be learnt about the actions of sex hormones on the arterial wall.

EXPERIMENTAL ARTERIAL DISEASE

The first experiments on the effects of sex hormones on blood and aortic cholesterol were reported in 1941. Administration of testosterone or oestradiol to cholesterol-fed rabbits caused a reduction in both blood and aortic cholesterol levels in female but not in male animals[1]. The hormones had no effect on rabbits fed a normal diet[2] or on ovariectomized rabbits fed normal or high-cholesterol diets[3]. It is notable that, in these experiments, oestrogens and androgens had the same protective effect, but only in female rabbits.

Many of the early investigations of the effect of exogenous oestrogens on experimental atherosclerosis used chickens as the experimental model. These were chosen because they develop arterial lesions which were considered to resemble human atherosclerosis. In one of the earliest reported studies[4] the implantation of diethylstilboestrol pellets into cockerels fed a normal diet resulted in hyperlipidaemia and the development of extensive lesions in the aorta after 6–7 months. These lesions consisted not only of lipids but also of cellular proliferation and connective tissue. This was the first time that hyperlipidaemia and aortic lesions had been produced in the absence of a high-cholesterol diet. The result was also the opposite to what might have been expected. The results were confirmed 2 years later in cockerels which were started on diethyl stilboestrol at a younger age to avoid the complicating effects of spontaneous lesions[5]. On both a normal- and a low-fat diet, oestrogen-treated birds developed marked hypercholesterolaemia and lesions in the thoracic aorta.

In contrast to the results of these experiments, it was later found that oral administration of oestradiol inhibited the development of atheromatous lesions in the coronary arteries of cockerels on high-cholesterol diets[6]. Oestradiol had no effect on aortic lesions. The major effect of oestradiol on plasma lipids was to increase lipid phosphorus, with little change in cholesterol. The protective effect of oestrogens could be partially or completely abolished by hypothyroidism[7] or by insulin[8]. Although in similar experiments testosterone slightly reduced plasma cholesterol levels, it had no effect on lesions in the aorta or coronary arteries[9]. It was concluded that oestrogens were the most important sex hormones in atherogenesis.

The effects of sex hormones on lipid and connective tissue responses have also been studied in other laboratory animals. Administration of oestradiol to castrated male and female rats resulted in an increase in lipid-containing lesions in the coronary arteries by 6 weeks but a decline in the lesions by 18 weeks. Testosterone had no effect[10]. On the other hand, oestradiol increased the degradation of collagen and elastin in the aortas of ovariectomized rats[11] while testosterone increased fibrous protein, elastin and collagen in the aortic wall of male rats[12]. Oestradiol, progesterone and testosterone all increased the glycosaminoglycan content of the aortas of hypophysectomized dogs but the different hormones acted in different parts of the aorta and had only a modest effect on the coronary arteries[13]. Oestrogens prevented aortic wall hypertrophy and reduced synthesis of collagen and elastin in male rats with experimental hypertension[14] but ethinyloestradiol, a synthetic oestrogen, caused intimal thickening with smooth muscle cells and elastic fibres in the aortas of female rats[15]. Chlormadinone acetate, a progestogen, alone or in combination with the oestrogen, had a variable effect on intimal thickening. Progestogen had a slight stimulatory effect in the hypertensive rats and less effect in the female rats. Endothelial permeability, studied by measuring the uptake of radiolabelled albumin, was increased by ethinyloestradiol in ovari-ectomized rats[16]. Increased permeability of the endothelium to plasma constituents is thought to be an early stage in the development of atherosclerosis. In pigeons, oestrogens decreased spontaneous arterial lesions[17,18]. Oestrogens also decreased the severity but not the prevalence of lesions in the coronary arteries of cholesterol-fed pigeons[19]. In pigeons fed a cholesterol-free diet, administration of conjugated equine oestrogen for 6 months resulted in an increase in aortic free cholesterol and a decrease in aortic cholesteryl esters[20]. Accumulation of cholesteryl esters is one of the features of spontaneous human atherosclerosis.

There has been only one report of the effect of sex hormones on lipids and atherosclerosis in subhuman primates[21]. In a series of experiments the effect of three different oestrogens was studied in the baboon, an animal whose physiological and pathological responses are more human-like than

THE EFFECTS OF SEX HORMONES

chickens, rats and rabbits. All the animals were fed high-fat diets, and they were given oestradiol, ethinyloestradiol or diethylstilboestrol. All were ovariectomized except one control group. Serum triglyceride and phospholipid were slightly elevated in the oestrogen-treated groups and the group with intact ovaries compared to ovariectomized untreated controls but cholesterol was unchanged. There was no consistent effect of oestrogen deficiency or replacement on the extent or quality of atherosclerotic lesions. These experiments thus showed no effects of oestrogen deficiency or oestrogen replacement therapy on serum lipid or lipoprotein concentrations or on atherosclerosis.

A different approach to the effect of oestrogens on experimental atherosclerosis has been prompted by the paradoxical hypolipidaemic effect of oestrogens in type III hyperlipidaemia in humans[22]. The lipoproteins which characterize this disorder are similar to those found in cholesterol-fed rabbits. Oestradiol markedly attenuated the rise in lipids in cholesterol-fed rabbits[23]. Within plasma cholesterol, the rise in LDL cholesterol remained unchanged while the rises in VLDL and IDL cholesterol were markedly attenuated (Table 12.1). Apolipoprotein composition in the oestrogen-treated cholesterol-fed rabbits resembled that in non-cholesterol-fed control animals. Aortic lesions and aortic

Table 12.1 Effect of oestrogen treatment on plasma lipids and lipoproteins, aortic lipids and aortic lesions in cholesterol-fed rabbits

	Cholesterol-fed untreated rabbits	Cholesterol-fed oestrogen-treated rabbits
Plasma lipids (mg/dl)		
Total cholesterol	825 ± 259*	331 ± 160
Total triglyceride	52 ± 32	16 ± 5
VLDL-C	374 ± 149*	63 ± 60
IDL-C	182 ± 126*	86 ± 50
LDL-C	100 ± 23	116 ± 75
HDL-C	20 ± 5	24 ± 10
Aortic lipids (g/100 g dry wt)		
Cholesterol	6.16 ± 1.55*	1.24 ± 0.44
Triglyceride	7.00 ± 1.62*	10.96 ± 5.57
Phospholipid	2.90 ± 0.55	1.38 ± 0.16
Aortic lesions (score 0-4)		
	3.13 ± 0.85*	0.13 ± 0.05

* Significant ($p < 0.05$) difference between groups
VLDL-C = very low-density lipoprotein cholesterol
IDL-C = intermediate-density lipoprotein cholesterol
LDL-C = low-density lipoprotein cholesterol
HDL-C = high-density lipoprotein cholesterol
(From Kushwaha and Hazzard 1981[23])

cholesterol and phospholipid content were much lower in the oestrogen-treated animals than in the untreated cholesterol-fed controls. Animals whose total plasma cholesterol was adjusted by dietary means to be the same as that in the oestrogen-treated cholesterol-fed rabbits had higher VLDL, lower LDL and similar HDL cholesterol levels and markedly greater aortic lesions. This suggests that the lipoprotein composition, rather than total or LDL cholesterol, was important in producing aortic lesions in these experiments. It was suggested that oestrogens accelerated the catabolism of VLDL remnants by the liver, perhaps by increasing the hepatic uptake of these particles[24]. The results of the experiments are consistent with the suggestion that remnants of triglyceride-rich lipoproteins are particularly atherogenic[25].

It is difficult to find a common theme in the results of the different experimental approaches to sex hormones and atherosclerosis. It seems clear that the results are influenced by the species of animal chosen, the artery studied, the composition of the diet and the type and route of administration of the oestrogen. In view of the great influence of these experimental variables on the results of the studies, their relevance to the effects of the administration of oestrogens to normal humans remains unclear.

SEX HORMONES AND THROMBOSIS

Among the vascular complications of oral contraceptives are venous thrombosis and pulmonary embolism. This suggests that sex hormones may influence the clotting process. Thrombosis may also have a role in the arterial complications of oral contraceptives as a thrombus superimposed on an atheromatous plaque may be the cause of an arterial occlusion. The formed elements of the blood, particularly platelets, may also contribute to the pathogenesis of the atheromatous lesion.

An early study of the effect of sex hormones on thrombosis used, as an experimental model, the effect of intravenous infusions of pooled dog sera on clotting in the renal veins of rats[26]. Ten times more serum was needed to induce clotting in females than in males. Ovariectomy reduced the level in females to that of males while treatment with conjugated oestrogens returned it to the normal female range. Testosterone also reduced the clotting threshold in normal females. Endocrine manipulation had little effect on clotting in males. The effect of sex hormones on experimental thrombogenesis has also been studied using a technique of inducing thrombosis by damaging rat aortic endothelium with an intra-arterial catheter[27,28]. Thrombogenesis was measured by the obstruction time of the cannula, the dry thrombus weight and the mortality rate. Thrombus weight and mortality were greater and obstruction time less in male than in female rats. In both sexes, thrombus weight and mortality increased and obstruction time decreased with increasing age. Testosterone increased thrombus formation in male and female rats while oestradiol marginally reduced thrombus formation in male rats only. The thrombogenic effects of testosterone were inhibited by an antiandrogen and by aspirin. The sex difference in thrombus formation in rats was also found in rabbits and in mice[29].

Sex hormones may influence thrombogenesis by actions on the constituents of the blood or on the vessel wall. Aggregation of platelets in response to ADP was ten times higher when they were obtained from male rats than female rats of the same age[30]. Castration of male rats decreased platelet aggregability, while ovariectomy increased the aggregation of platelets from female rats. Similarly treatment with testosterone *in vivo* or *in vitro* increased the aggregability of platelets from female rats. The effect of different androgens on platelet aggregation was directly related to their androgenicity, and testosterone's effect was abolished by oestradiol and by an antiandrogen. Aggregation in response to ADP of platelets from male rabbits was depressed by treatment with the oestrogens diethylstilboestrol, oestradiol or conjugated equine oestrogens[31]. Oestradiol had a similar effect on platelets from female rabbits. The oestrogens had no effect on aggregation of platelets in response to collagen nor on platelet adhesiveness. A progestogen had no effect on platelet aggregation or adhesiveness. Sex differences in human platelet aggregation have also been described[32].

One of the most important inhibitors of platelet aggregation is prostacyclin, a product of arachidonic acid metabolism in the vascular endothelium. In rats, treatment with the oestrogen ethinyloestradiol increased prostacyclin-like activity in the aorta, while the progestogen norethisterone had no effect[33]. Neither hormone altered prostacyclin-like activity in the inferior vena cava. Another oestrogen, oestradiol, increased prostacyclin production in cultured rat aortic smooth muscle cells[34,35] and in whole rat aorta[36] but had no effect on thromboxane production by platelets[36]. Thromboxane is a product of arachidonic acid metabolism in the platelet and is a potent promoter of platelet aggregation.

The experimental evidence on the effect of sex and sex hormones on the clotting process is remarkably consistent. Male sex is associated with greater thrombogenesis than female sex, and male sex hormones increase thrombus formation. Androgens increase platelet aggregability while oestrogens have the opposite effect. Oestrogens also increase prostacyclin formation and activity in the arterial wall. The evidence that the female sex and its hormones inhibits thrombus formation is consistent with the lesser incidence of vascular disease in women, but is not consistent with the association of oestrogen-containing drugs with thromboembolic and arterial disease.

SEX HORMONES AND CULTURED ARTERIAL CELLS

Both arterial endothelial and smooth muscle cells are important in the pathogenesis of atherosclerosis. Loss of endothelial integrity is probably a very early stage in atherogenesis, while proliferation of smooth muscle cells in the intima is the earliest identifiable lesion. An effect of sex hormones on proliferation of these cells may thus have important implications in atherogenesis.

There have only been two studies of the direct effects of sex hormones on the growth of cultured arterial cells[35,37]. Endothelial cells were cultured from human umbilical vein and smooth muscle cells from rat aorta[37]. Proliferation was studied by measuring the incorporation of radiolabelled thymidine into DNA. Ethinyloestradiol, oestrone and oestriol had no effect on DNA synthesis in either type of cell (Figure 12.1). Oestradiol had no effect on cell numbers when added to cultured rat aortic smooth muscle cells[35]. These results contrast with the stimulating effect of oestrogens and androgens on the proliferation of an established mouse fibroblast cell line[38]. An indirect effect of sex hormones on arterial cells is possible as serum from women taking oral contraceptives stimulates proliferation[39] and sterol synthesis[40] in cultured human arterial smooth muscle cells. The individual steroid components of the drug had no effect on the latter process. It has also been shown that an oestrogen-induced protein from rat tissues

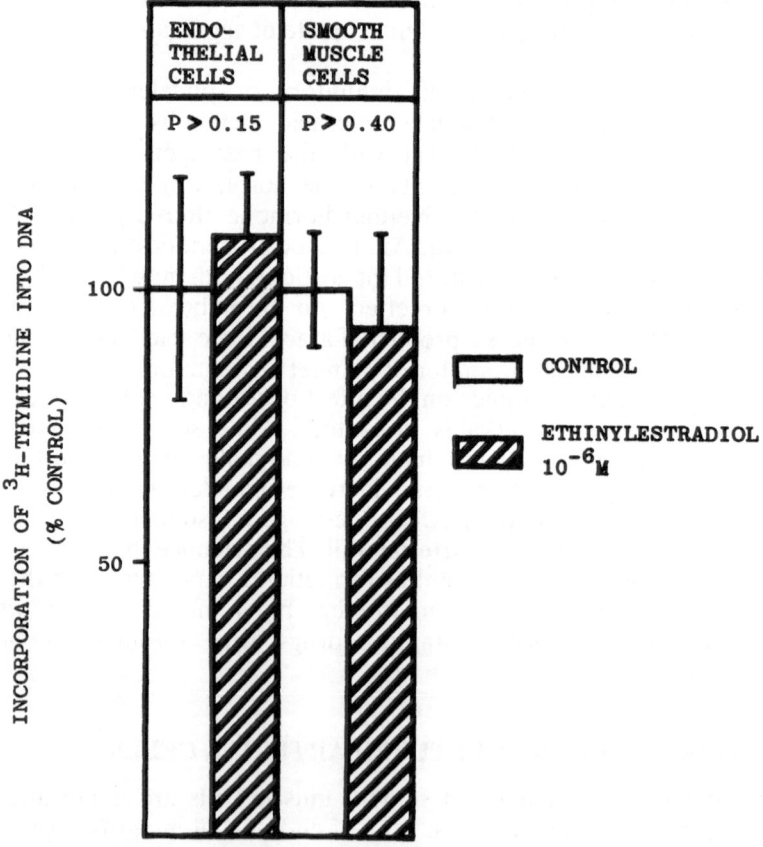

Figure 12.1 Effect of ethinyloestradiol (10^{-6} mmol/l) on DNA synthesis in cultured human umbilical venous endothelial cells and rat aortic smooth muscle cells. (Data from Taggart and Stout, 1980[37])

stimulates DNA synthesis in cultured fibroblasts[41] and enhances growth in a number of hormone-responsive tumour cells[42]. The pure hormone had no effect on either process.

Studies of the effect of sex hormones on arterial cell growth and lipid metabolism are sparse and the results are at present unhelpful. The possibility that sex hormones induce the formation of a growth factor is worth further study.

RECEPTORS FOR SEX HORMONES IN THE ARTERIAL WALL

Hormones interact with their target cells by means of specific cell receptors. For peptide hormones the receptors are on the cell membrane, but steroid hormones interact with cytoplasmic receptors. Receptors for several sex hormones have been identified in arterial cells.

Earlier studies showed that radiolabelled oestradiol injected into humans is found in blood vessels as well as other tissues[43] and that arterial tissue is able to metabolize oestrogens and androgens[44]. Labelled oestradiol is also found within cardiac muscle cells[45]. More specifically oestradiol binding sites have been identified in cultured rabbit aortic endothelial cells[46] in cultured rat aortic smooth muscle cells[47] and in smooth muscle cells of dog coronary arteries[48]. Radiolabelled testosterone and oestradiol injected into baboons was found in the nuclei of arterial endothelial and smooth muscle cells confirming the presence of sex hormone receptors in these cells[49]. Androgen binding has also been identified in smooth muscle cells of the anterior and middle cerebral arteries of the rat[50]. Cytoplasmic androgen receptors have recently been biochemically identified in the aorta of the baboon[51].

There is thus consistent evidence that arterial endothelial and smooth muscle cells have receptors for both oestrogens and androgens. The physiological significance of these receptors is not clear, as there is little evidence that sex hormones have direct activities on arterial cells. There are other examples of the presence of hormone receptors in cells that appear resistant to the actions of the respective hormones[52]. Further knowledge of endocrine physiology is needed to explain these apparent contradictions. In the meantime, the significance of sex hormone receptors in arterial cells in the pathogenesis of atherosclerosis must remain an open question.

CONCLUSIONS

It is difficult to draw conclusions from the conflicting results of studies on the effects of sex hormones on the arterial wall. The animal species used, the artery studied, the diet, the lipid pattern produced, and the type of sex hormone studied all seem to influence the findings. Despite the presence of oestrogen and androgen receptors there is no evidence that sex hormones have a direct effect on proliferation or lipid synthesis in arterial cells. The direct effect of hormones on connective tissue metabolism of cultured arterial cells have not been studied. The possibility that oestrogens act indirectly on arterial cells by means of a factor produced elsewhere in the body has been suggested but not fully explored. Oestrogens inhibit the development of vascular disease by increasing the production of prostacyclin in the arterial wall. Oestrogens also inhibit coagulation and platelet aggregation while androgens have the opposite effect. Apart from this mechanism, it has to be concluded that the effects of sex hormones on experimental atherosclerosis in the intact animal are likely to be secondary to effects on lipid metabolism. The fact that insulin can overcome the protective effect of oestrogens in cholesterol-fed chickens is of interest in view of the fact that diabetes overcomes the protective effect of the female sex in human atherosclerosis.

References

1. Ludden, J. B., Bruger, M. and Wright, I. S. (1942). Experimental atherosclerosis. IV. Effect of testosterone propionate and estradiol dipropionate on experimental atherosclerosis in rabbits. *Arch. Pathol.*, **33**, 58
2. Ludden, J. B., Bruger, M. and Wright, I. S. (1941). Effect of testosterone propionate and estradiol dipropionate on the cholesterol content of the blood and aorta of rabbits. *Endocrinology*, **28**, 999
3. Bruger, M., Wright, I. S. and Wiland, J. (1943). Experimental atherosclerosis. V. Effect of testosterone propionate and estradiol dipropionate on the cholesterol content of the blood and the aorta in castrate female rabbits. *Arch. Pathol.*, **36**, 612
4. Lindsay, S., Lorenz, F. W., Entenman, C. and Chaikoff, I. L. (1946). Production of atheromatosis in the aorta of the chicken by administration of diethylstilbesterol. *Proc. Soc. Exp. Biol. Med.*, **62**, 315
5. Horlick, L. and Katz, L. N. (1948). The effect of diethylstilbestrol on blood lipids and the development of atherosclerosis in chickens on a normal and low fat diet. *J. Lab. Clin. Med.*, **33**, 733
6. Pick, R., Stamler, J., Rodbard, S. and Katz, L. N. (1952). The inhibition of coronary atherosclerosis by estrogens in cholesterol-fed chicks. *Circulation*, **6**, 276
7. Pick, R., Stamler, J. and Katz, L. N. (1957). Effects of hypothyroidism on estrogen-induced inhibition of coronary atherogenesis in cholesterol-fed cockerels. *Circ. Res.*, **5**, 510
8. Stamler, J., Pick, R. and Katz, L. N. (1960). Effect of insulin in the induction and regression of atherosclerosis in the chick. *Circ. Res.*, **8**, 572
9. Pick, R., Stamler, J., Rodbard, S. and Katz, L. N. (1959). Effects of testosterone and castration on cholesteremia and atherogenesis in chicks on high fat, high cholesterol diets. *Circ. Res.*, **7**, 202
10. Moskowitz, M. S., Moskowitz, A. A., Bradford, W. L. and Wissler, R. W. (1956). Changes in serum lipids and coronary arteries of the rat in response to estrogen. *Arch. Pathol.*, **61**, 245
11. Fischer, G. M. (1972). In vivo effects of estradiol on collagen and elastin dynamics in rat aorta. *Endocrinology*, **91**, 1227
12. Wolinsky, H. (1972). Effects of androgen treatment on the male rat aorta. *J. Clin. Invest.*, **51**, 2552
13. Sirek, O. V., Sirek, A. and Fikar, K. (1977). The effect of sex hormones on glycosaminoglycan content of canine aorta and coronary arteries. *Atherosclerosis*, **27**, 227
14. Wolinsky, H. (1972). Effects of estrogen and progestogen treatment on the response of the aorta of male rats to hypertension. *Circ. Res.*, **30**, 341
15. Gammal, E. B. (1976). Intimal thickening in arteries of rats treated with synthetic sex hormones. *Br. J. Exp. Pathol.*, **57**, 248
16. Gammal, E. B. and Zuk, A. (1980). Effect of ethinyl estradiol on endothelial permeability to ^{125}I-labelled albumin in female rats. *Exp. Mol. Pathol.*, **32**, 91
17. Souadjian, J. V., Kottke, B. A. and Titus, J. L. (1968). Estrogen effects on spontaneous atherosclerosis. Experimental studies in white carneau pigeon. *Arch. Pathol.*, **85**, 463

18. Hanash, K. A., Kottke, B. A., Greene, L. F. and Titus, J. L. (1972). Effects of conjugated estrogens on spontaneous atherosclerosis in pigeons. *Arch. Pathol.*, **93**, 184

19. Prichard, R. W., Clarkson, T. B. and Lofland, H. B. (1966). Estrogen in pigeon atherosclerosis. Estradiol valerate effects at several dose levels on cholesterol-fed male white carneau pigeons. *Arch. Pathol.*, **82**, 15

20. Subbiah, M. T. R. and Dicke, B. A. (1977). Effect of estrogens on the concentration and composition of arterial sterols and steryl esters in male white carneau pigeons. *Atherosclerosis*, **27**, 59

21. McGill, H. C., Jr, Axelrod, L. R., McMahan, C. A., Wigodsky, H. S. and Mott, G. E. (1977). Estrogens and experimental atherosclerosis in the baboon (*Papio cynocephalus*). *Circulation*, **56**, 657

22. Kushwaha, R. S., Hazzard, W. R., Gagne, C., Chait, A. and Albers, J. J. (1977). Type III hyperlipoproteinemia: paradoxical hypolipidemic response to estrogen. *Ann. Intern. Med.*, **87**, 517

23. Kushwaha, R. S. and Hazzard, W. R. (1981). Exogenous estrogens attenuate dietary hypercholesterolemia and atherosclerosis in the rabbit. *Metabolism*, **30**, 359

24. Floren, C.-H., Kushwaha, R. S., Hazzard, W. R. and Albers, J. J. (1981). Estrogen-induced increase in uptake of cholesterol-rich very low density lipoproteins in perfused rabbit liver. *Metabolism*, **30**, 367

25. Zilversmit, D. B. (1973). A proposal linking atherosclerosis to the interaction of endothelial lipoprotein lipase with triglyceride-rich lipoproteins. *Circ. Res.*, **33**, 633

26. Amos, S., Odake, K., Ambrus, C. M. and Ambrus, J. L. (1969). Effect of sex hormones on the serum-induced thrombosis phenomenon. *Proc. Natl. Acad. Sci., USA*, **62**, 150

27. Uzunova, A., Ramey, E. and Ramwell, P. W. (1976). Effect of testosterone, sex and age on experimentally induced arterial thrombosis. *Nature (London)*, **261**, 712

28. Uzunova, A. D., Ramey, E. R. and Ramwell, P. W. (1978). Gonadal hormones and pathogenesis of occlusive arterial thrombosis. *Am. J. Physiol.*, **234**, H454

29. Uzunova, A. D., Ramey, E. R. and Ramwell, P. W. (1977). Arachidonate-induced thrombosis in mice: effects of gender or testosterone and estradiol administration. *Prostaglandins*, **13**, 995

30. Johnson, M., Ramey, E. and Ramwell, P. W. (1977). Androgen-mediated sensitivity in platelet aggregation. *Am. J. Physiol.*, **232**, H381

31. Mitchell, H. C. and Williams, M. A. (1974). Effect of estrogens and a progestogen on platelet adhesiveness and aggregation in rabbits. *J. Lab. Clin. Med.*, **83**, 79

32. Johnson, M., Ramey, E. and Ramwell, P. W. (1975). Sex and age differences in human platelet aggregation. *Nature (London)*, **253**, 355

33. Karpati, L., Chow, F. P. R., Woollard, M. L., Hutton, R. A. and Dandona, P. (1980). Prostacyclin-like activity in the female rat thoracic aorta and the inferior vena cava after ethinyloestradiol and norethisterone. *Clin. Sci.*, **59**, 369

34. Chang, W., Nakao, J., Orimo, H. and Murota, S. (1980). Stimulation of prostacyclin biosynthetic activity by estradiol in rat aortic smooth muscle cells in culture. *Biochim. Biophys. Acta*, **619**, 107

35. Chang, W.-C., Nakao, J., Orimo, H. and Murota, S.-I. (1980). Stimulation of prostaglandin cyclooxygenase and prostacyclin synthetase activities by estradiol in rat aortic smooth muscle cells. *Biochim. Biophys. Acta*, **620**, 472

36. Chang, W.-C., Nakao, J., Neichi, T., Orimo, H. and Murota, S.-I. (1981). Effects of estradiol on the metabolism of arachidonic acid by aortas and platelets in rats. *Biochim. Biophys. Acta*, **664**, 291

37. Taggart, H. and Stout, R. W. (1980). Control of DNA synthesis in cultured vascular endothelial and smooth muscle cells – response to serum, platelet-deficient serum, lipid-free serum, insulin and oestrogens. *Atherosclerosis*, **37**, 549

38. Jung-Testas, I. and Baulieu, E.-E. (1979). Effects of sex steroids and anti-hormones on growth adhesiveness and receptors of L-929 cells cultured in serum-containing and serum-free media. *Exp. Cell Res.*, **119**, 75

39. Bagdade, J. D. and Cruz, R. (1977). 'The Pill' and the pathogenesis of atherosclerosis: serum factors stimulate arterial smooth muscle cell and fibroblast proliferation. *Circulation*, **55/56**, suppl. III-101

40. Subbaiah, P. V. and Bagdade, J. D. (1980). Oral contraceptive steroids and

atherosclerosis: lipogenesis in human arterial smooth muscle cells and dermal fibroblasts in presence of lipoprotein-deficient serum from oral contraceptive users. *Artery*, **6**, 437

41. King, R. J. B., Kaye, A. M. and Shodell, M. J. (1977). Co-purification of an oestrogen-induced protein from rat uterus and a factor able to stimulate DNA synthesis in cultured cells. *Exp. Cell Res.*, **109**, 1

42. Sirbasku, D. A. (1978). Estrogen induction of growth factors specific for hormone-responsive mammary, pituitary and kidney tumor cells. *Proc. Natl. Acad. Sci., USA*, **75**, 3786

43. Malinow, M. R., Moguilevsky, J. A., Lema, B. and Bur, G. E. (1963). Vascular and extravascular radioactivity after the injection of estradiol 6, 7H^3 in the human being. *J. Clin. Endocrinol. Metab.*, **23**, 206

44. Chobanian, A. V., Brecher, P. I., Lille, R. D. and Wotiz, H. H. (1968). Metabolism of sex hormones in the aortic wall. *J. Lipid Res.*, **9**, 701

45. Stumpf, W. E., Sar, M. and Aumuller, G. (1977). The heart: a target organ for estradiol. *Science*, **196**, 319

46. Colburn, P. and Buonassisi, V. (1978). Estrogen-binding sites in endothelial cell cultures. *Science*, **201**, 817

47. Nakao, J., Chang, W.-C., Murota, S.-I. and Orimo, H. (1981). Estradiol-binding sites in rat aortic smooth muscle cells in culture. *Atherosclerosis*, **38**, 75

48. Harder, D. R. and Coulson, P. B. (1979). Estrogen receptors and effects of estrogen on membrane electrical properties of coronary vascular smooth muscle. *J. Cell Physiol.*, **100**, 375

49. McGill, H. C., Jr and Sheridan, P. J. (1981). Nuclear uptake of sex steroid hormones in the cardiovascular system of the baboon. *Circ. Res.*, **48**, 238

50. Sheridan, P. J. and Buchanan, J. M. (1980). The effects of opiates on androgen binding in the forebrain of the rat. *Int. J. Fertil.*, **25**, 36

51. Lin, A. L., McGill, H. C., Jr and Shain, S. A. (1981). Hormone receptors of the baboon cardiovascular system. Biochemical characterization of aortic cytoplasmic androgen receptors. *Arteriosclerosis*, **1**, 257

52. Stout, R. W. (1982). Hormone–endothelial interactions. In Cryer, A. (ed.) *Biochemical Interactions at the Endothelium*. (Amsterdam: Elsevier/North Holland; in press)

13
Sex hormones and atherosclerosis – conclusions

It is difficult to draw conclusions about the relationship of sex hormones to atherosclerosis. There is no doubt that in parts of the world where atherosclerosis is common, cardiovascular disease is more prevalent in younger men than in women of the same age. Whether this is due to acceleration of atherosclerosis in males or protection against athero- sclerosis in females is unclear. Nor is it clear that the differences are related to hormone secretion. The fact that the difference in incidence in males and females decreases after the menopause may suggest endocrine mechanisms, but other factors may also be involved.

The association of exogenous sex hormones with atherosclerosis is not entirely consistent with the male–female differential. Although the type and dose of hormone used and the hormonal status of the recipient are all important, it seems clear that oestrogens can predispose to cardiovascular disease. It is also clear that oestrogens do not protect men or postmenopausal women from atherosclerosis. Thus, study of the effects of exogenous sex hormones on atherosclerosis has not helped to resolve the questions on the association of endogenous sex hormone secretion and cardiovascular disease.

While lipid and lipoprotein levels in males and females in general parallel incidence rates of atherosclerosis, the effects of exogenous sex hormones on lipid metabolism are not consistent with these hormones being responsible for the differences. The results of studies of the effects of sex hormones on experimental atherosclerosis are also confusing, and there is no evidence that sex hormones have a direct effect on the arterial wall. An effect on connective tissue metabolism is the most likely but is unproven by direct experiment. There is, however, evidence that the female sex and oestrogens are associated with reduced coagulation and increased synthesis of prostacyclin.

Among the important unanswered questions about sex hormones and atherosclerosis are the following:

(1) Is the difference in cardiovascular disease incidence in younger men

and women due to a promoting factor in men or a protective factor in women?

(2) Is the sex difference in cardiovascular disease due to disease of the arterial wall or to thrombosis? Autopsy studies indicate that disease of the arterial wall is involved but new studies using modern techniques are needed.

(3) Do sex hormones cause the production of another factor which has direct actions on the arterial wall?

(4) Do male and female arterial cells respond differently to stimuli including risk factors for atherosclerosis? Cell culture studies should answer this question.

(5) What is the role of changes in carbohydrate metabolism and insulin secretion induced by sex hormones in the development of atherosclerosis? Little attention has been paid to this aspect of sex hormone action. It is possible that changes in glucose and insulin are a mechanism linking sex hormones to atherosclerosis.

THYROID

14
Thyroid function and atherosclerosis

HYPOTHYROIDISM AND ATHEROSCLEROSIS

There have been many observations of heart disease in association with hypothyroidism. Most of these have been isolated case reports and have been somewhat anecdotal. The early reports are reviewed by Smyth and Arbor[1]. Much attention has been paid to the difficulties of managing hypothyroidism in the patient with heart disease as thyroid replacement may worsen angina or precipitate cardiac failure in the predisposed patient[2].

One of the problems of assessing the role of hypothyroidism in atherosclerosis is the fact that treatment is usually instituted as soon as the hypothyroid state is identified. This problem was overcome in a study of eight patients who were rendered hypothyroid therapeutically for treatment of angina pectoris or congestive cardiac failure caused by rheumatic heart disease or cor pulmonale[3]. The patients were hypothyroid for 1–13 years. All had elevated cholesterol levels compared to pre-treatment values, and some had grossly elevated levels (over 400 mg/dl). Despite this, excess coronary atherosclerosis was not found, and none of the patients had complete occlusions of any coronary arteries. The authors quote a study of 209 cases of myxoedema described in 1888 by the Committee of the Clinical Society of London. At that time, before any effective treatment of myxoedema was known, excessive atherosclerosis was not found. Further studies quoted show that extensive atherosclerosis is not universal in subjects with cretinism or juvenile myxoedema. Thus, this study does not support a role for either hypothyroidism or hyper-cholesterolaemia in atherosclerosis.

Evidence of an association between hypothyroidism and coronary artery disease comes from a post-mortem study from Finland showing that goitre was commoner and the average weight of the thyroid gland was heavier in patients who died from coronary artery disease than in those who died from other causes[4]. Another post-mortem study (Table 14.1) showed a higher frequency of severe coronary atherosclerosis in subjects with untreated

157

myxoedema compared to controls[5]. In a clinical study by the same authors, electrocardiographic evidence of myocardial ischaemia and other abnormalities were more common in the hypothyroid patients (Table 14.2).

Table 14.1 Autopsy coronary atherosclerosis and myocardial infarctions in hypothyroid subjects and controls (percentages)[5]

	Hypothyroid	*Controls*
Coronary atherosclerosis		
degree 0	4	40
1	12	14
2	84	46
Myocardial infarct	24	6

Table 14.2 ECG abnormalities in hypothyroid patients and controls (percentages)[5]

	Hypothyroid	*Controls*
Normal	5	29
Ischaemia	11	0
Infarct	16	14
Left ventricular strain	16	11
Disturbances of A-V conduction	18	2

There appears to have been only one systematic autopsy study of coronary artery disease and myxoedema and this was retrospective[6]. From the records of the Massachusetts General Hospital, adult white women with a pathological diagnosis of thyroid atrophy and a clinical and laboratory diagnosis of hypothyroidism were studied. The records were reviewed for heart weight, left ventricular thickness, myocardial infarction, degree of atherosclerosis of the coronary arteries and cause of death. Hypertension was diagnosed from the clinical records of blood pressure and pathological evidence of hypertension. Random controls were also selected from the records. The myxoedema patients had much more severe coronary artery disease than the controls. Although the frequency of hypertension was no different in the myxoedema and control groups, the difference between the hypothyroid group and the controls was related entirely to the increase in coronary artery disease in the myxoedema patients with hypertension – the hypertensives had twice as much coronary artery narrowing as control hypertensives. On the other hand, hypothyroid normotensives had no increase in coronary narrowing compared to control normotensives. Hypothyroid patients had an average coronary narrowing of greater than 75% against an average coronary narrowing of less than 50% in control patients with hypertension. These findings suggest that it is only in the presence of hypertension that hypothyroidism contributes to increased coronary narrowing. It is not clear whether the subjects with myxoedema were treated with thyroid replacement or how adequate the treatment was, but the implication from the presentation of the data is that the patients were treated. Serum cholesterol levels were elevated in the majority of hypothyroid subjects, in some instances, markedly so.

Because of the lipid lowering effects of thyroid hormone, dextro-thyroxine has been used in a large trial on the secondary prevention of myocardial infarction[7]. Dextrothyroxine is a less active isomer of the naturally occurring hormone, levothyroxine. Early in the trial, dextro-thyroxine had to be discontinued in a group of patients who had frequent ventricular ectopic beats at the beginning of the study as the mortality was high in this group. After a mean follow-up period of 36 months the dextrothyroxine group was found to have an 18.4% higher mortality rate than the placebo group and the drug was stopped. The excess mortality occurred particularly in those with a history of complicated myocardial infarction, angina, raised blood pressure or ECG conduction defects and occurred despite a fall in both cholesterol and triglyceride. The mechanism of the adverse effect is unknown.

Overall the evidence of a close link between hypothyroidism and atherosclerosis is not convincing. If hypothyroidism has a role in atherogenesis, it appears to be facilitatory rather than causal, increasing the effects of other factors in the pathogenesis of atherosclerosis. It may be that some other variable in addition to hypothyroidism and accompanying hypercholesterolaemia is necessary to produce atherosclerosis and that this factor is present only in some patients. Congenital or surgically induced hypothyroidism may have a different association with atherosclerosis than hypothyroidism which occurs spontaneously in adults and which has an autoimmune basis.

AUTOIMMUNE THYROIDITIS AND CORONARY HEART DISEASE

A number of studies, chiefly from Bastenie's group in Belgium, have suggested that preclinical hypothyroidism, diagnosed by the presence of thyroid antibodies in subjects with normal thyroid function, is associated with coronary artery disease. Subjects who were clinically euthyroid were studied for the presence of thyroglobulin antibodies and for the presence of clinical and ECG signs of myocardial ischaemia[8]. It was found that 22% of patients with thyroglobulin antibodies had evidence of coronary artery disease compared with 12% of patients without antibodies – a statistically significant difference (Table 14.3). Conversely, 30% of patients over 50 years of age with coronary disease had thyroglobulin antibodies compared to 17% without coronary disease. A retrospective study of post-mortem records showed that lymphocytic infiltration of the thyroid was much

Table 14.3 Thyroglobulin antibodies (TGA) in controls and in patients with coronary artery disease (CAD) (percentages)[8]

With TGA	
Patients over 50 without CAD	17
Patients over 50 with CAD	30
With CAD	
Patients without TGA	12
Patients with TGA	22

commoner in both males and females with myocardial infarction than in those without. In a later study, the association of thyroid antibodies and myocardial infarction was studied in 400 women and 400 men[9]. The subjects were admitted to hospital for non-thyroid related diseases and thus were not a random selection of the population. The median age of the women was 64 and that of the men was 60. In the female patients with asymptomatic thyroiditis, an increased prevalence of myocardial infarction, obesity, diabetes and hypertension was found compared with the non-thyroiditis controls. In the male population, a significant association was found between thyroiditis and obesity, diabetes and hypertension but not between thyroiditis and myocardial infarction. Thryoiditis increased the prevalence of coronary heart disease (CHD) in females without obesity, hypertension or diabetes but had less effect when these conditions were present. In women but not men, thyroiditis was associated with raised serum cholesterol levels. These data suggest that thyroid autoimmunity may be associated with coronary artery disease, particularly in females of this age. The relationship of obesity, hypertension and diabetes with thyroid antibodies and coronary artery disease remains unclear. A further study of asymptomatic autoimmune thyroiditis and CHD[10] used two cohorts of men from Finland: one from eastern Finland, where the coronary heart disease incidence is high, and the other from southwestern Finland where CHD incidence is half that in the east. A third group of subjects came from Yugoslavia where CHD morbidity is very low. In Yugoslavia, thyroid antibodies were uncommon and no relationship between CHD and the various measures of thyroid function was found. In the Finnish studies, the association between thyroid antibodies and CHD reached statistical significance in the west Finland cohort although in both areas 31% of men with thyroid antibodies had CHD. High TSH levels were also found in subjects with CHD. A prospective study in a Finnish cohort was carried out between 1969 and 1974. Whereas in the west 29%, and in the east 41% of men without thyroid antibodies in 1969 had or acquired CHD during the 5-year interval between the studies, 53% and 63% respectively of those with thyroid antibodies in 1969 had CHD by 1974. All subjects in this study were men, and the average ages were 63–65. A study of familial hyperlipidaemia in survivors of myocardial infarction in Seattle, USA found elevated TSH levels in five of 18 hyperlipidaemic women over age 60, and in a small number of the remaining hyperlipidaemic subjects[11]. Hypertriglyceridaemia was the lipid abnormality most closely associated with high TSH levels.

A different population survey from Finland failed to confirm the association of symptomless autoimmune thyroiditis in CHD[12]. This survey, which used 3569 subjects aged 30–59 years – part of a total community study, demonstrated the well-known association of hypertension and hypercholesterolaemia with CHD. However, there was no difference in TSH or PBI levels between coronary patients and controls and no association between thyroglobulin antibodies and the frequency of CHD. The study used a rather younger group of subjects than those in the Belgian studies. In an English community survey there was no association between ischaemic heart disease and thyroid antibodies or raised TSH levels in males[13]. In females there was no relation between thyroid antibodies or TSH levels and the more objective criteria of ischaemic heart disease (Tables 14.4 and 14.5). However, there was a weak association between these measures of thyroid function and cardiovascular symptoms and minor ECG changes. The significance of this observation is doubtful as a study of the same subjects 4 years later showed that the association had disappeared [14].

Table 14.4 Ischaemic heart disease and lipids in relation to autoimmune thyroiditis in an English community survey[13]

	Thyroid antibodies in males		Thyroid antibodies in females	
	Present	Absent	Present	Absent
History of IHD (%)	7.5	7.7	5.4	4.5
Possible MI (%)	5.0	5.5	5.4	3.7
Major ECG changes (%)	5.0	4.6	7.4	4.2
Cholesterol (mmol/l)	5.9 ± 0.18	5.8 ± 0.03	6.4 ± 0.12	6.2 ± 0.04*
Triglyceride (mmol/l)	1.52 ± 0.13	1.46 ± 0.03	1.15 ± 0.05	1.12 ± 0.02

* $p < 0.05$; remaining differences not significant
ECG = electrocardiograph
IHD = ischaemic heart disease
MI = myocardial infarction

Evidence of an association between autoimmune thyroiditis and CHD is conflicting. However, there is enough suggestive data to justify further studies, preferably of the prospective type. The mechanism of any association is unclear. It has been suggested that hypercholesterolaemia may occur in preclinical myxoedema[15] although the association has not been confirmed. Raised TSH levels are common in subjects with circulating thyroglobulin antibodies[16] and TSH may influence fat metabolism. An autoimmune mechanism of atherosclerosis is possible. The relation of the

Table 14.5   Ischaemic heart disease and lipids in relation to TSH levels in an English community survey[13]

	TSH (mU/l) males		TSH (mU/l) females	
	⩾ 6	< 6	⩾ 6	< 6
History of IHD (%)	11.4	7.7	7.2	4.2
Possible MI (%)	5.7	5.5	8.2	3.6*
Major ECG changes (%)	8.6	4.5	5.2	4.6
Cholesterol (mmol/l)	5.83 ± 0.15	5.80 ± 0.03	6.55 ± 0.15	6.14± 0.03*
Triglyceride (mmol/l)	1.56 ± 0.17	1.46 ± 0.03	1.22 ± 0.06	1.12 ± 0.02

* $p < 0.05$; remaining differences not significant
TSH = thyroid-stimulating hormone; other abbreviations as in Table 14.4

autoimmune thyroiditis to other diseases including diabetes must also be considered. An Australian study of 400 diabetics, 200 insulin-dependent and 200 non-insulin-dependent, and 400 matched controls, showed a high prevalence of antithyroid antibodies in the diabetics[17], most evident in young female diabetics. In contrast to the normal increase in prevalence of autoantibodies among ageing non-diabetics, antibody prevalence fell with age among diabetics. It was suggested that this may be because the presence of thyroid antibodies is associated with decreased survival in diabetics. Insulin-dependent diabetics with long-term diabetes had a 44% prevalence of thyrogastric antibodies compared with a 5% prevalence in the control group. In female diabetics there was a particularly strong association of thyroid antibodies with vascular disease. The highest prevalence · of thyrogastric antibodies was in the group of young diabetics with long-term insulin-dependent diabetes who in addition showed a high prevalence of vascular disease. It was also suggested in this study that the high prevalence of thyrogastric antibodies in insulin-dependent diabetics under the age of 40 years could be evidence of an advance by some 20 years of the ageing process in the diabetics. Thus, thyrogastric antibodies have wide implications and an association with vascular disease may not be direct but may be related to other factors. The relevance of autoantibodies in cardiovascular disease had been shown in the Busselton, Western Australia, study[18,19]. In a study of a number of different antibodies, it was found that thyrogastric antibodies were associated with angina, cerebrovascular disease and smoking. Thyrogastric autoimmunity had a strong genetic component which was linked to juvenile onset diabetes mellitus and possibly to vascular disease. The associations were particularly strong in men.

It is unlikely that autoimmune thyroiditis is secondary to vascular disease, but it is not clear that there is a causal link between thyroiditis and coronary artery disease[20]. As a link between hypothyroidism and atherosclerosis is by no means certain, it would be premature to suggest that minor abnormalities in thyroid function are causally linked to coronary artery disease. Possible harmful effects of ci culating immune complexes, or the association of autoimmunity with other metabolic abnormalities, including diabetes, are potential mechanisms which are worthy of further exploration.

POSSIBLE MECHANISMS OF ATHEROSCLEROSIS IN HYPOTHYROIDISM

Hypertension

There have been a number of suggestions that hypertension is common in hypothyroidism[21]. This would be surprising in view of the depressant effect of thyroid hormone deficiency on myocardial performance. The diagnosis of hypothyroidism in the study quoted would not be consistent with modern criteria. An autopsy study has suggested that atherosclerosis is only common in hypothyroid subjects who are also hypertensive[6]. However, there was no suggestion of a link between thyroid deficiency and hypertension.

Platelet and haemostatic abnormalities

A small study has shown decreased platelet adhesiveness in hypothyroidism and increased adhesiveness in hyperthyroidism, both returning towards normal with treatment of the thyroid disorder[22]. Haemostatic abnormalities with a tendency to prolonged bleeding have also been described in hypothyroidism[23]. These abnormalities included a prolonged activated partial thromboplastin time and reduced platelet factor 3 activity.

Thyroid hormones and arterial cells

Athough thyroid ablation has been used in combination with high-fat diets in studies on experimental atherosclerosis, there has been little published work on the effect of thyroid hormones on cultured arterial endothelial or smooth muscle cells. Tri-iodothyronine (T_3) had no effect on proliferation of cultured rat aortic smooth muscle cells[24]. However, in the same cells T_3 in increasing concentrations progressively increased the formation of prostacyclin. Prostacyclin is synthesized from arachidonic acid and is a potent vasodilator and inhibitor of platelet aggregation. While these experiments do not directly demonstrate that thyroid deficiency is associated with decreased prostacyclin synthesis, such a possibility exists. Hydrolase activities in the aorta of thyroidectomized rats were decreased compared to controls, but not to the same extent as in kidney and liver[25]. Hydrolase activity in liver and kidney more closely reflected the fractional clearance rate of low-density lipoproteins in the hypothyroid animals. It was suggested that the special vulnerability of vascular tissue to lipid deposition is a consequence of lack of synchronization of the metabolic responses of arterial smooth muscle cells to the overall metabolic load placed on this tissue by lipoproteins and haemodynamic factors.

CONCLUSIONS

The role of abnormalities of thyroid hormone secretion in atherosclerosis is unclear. It is unlikely to become clearer as treatment of the disorder is instituted without delay and there are important indications for treatment other than the prevention of atherosclerosis. It is likely that any association between hypothyroidism and atherosclerosis is secondary to the effects of thyroid deficiency on lipoprotein metabolism. In the majority of cases this is returned to normal by thyroid replacement therapy, and where it is not, some other cause of hyperlipidaemia usually coexists. The possibility of a widespread immunological disorder with associated autoimmune thyroiditis, atherosclerosis[26] and other disorders including diabetes mellitus is worthy of further study.

References

1. Smyth, C. J. and Arbor A. (1938). Angina pectoris and myocardial infarction as complications of myxedema. *Am. Heart J.*, **15**, 652
2. Levine, H. D. (1980). Compromise therapy in the patient with angina pectoris and hypothyroidism. *Am. J. Med.*, **69**, 411
3. Blumgart, H. L., Freedberg, A. S. and Kurland, G. S. (1953). Hypercholesterolemia, myxedema and atherosclerosis. *Am. J. Med.*, **14**, 665
4. Uotila, U., Raekallio, J. and Ehrnrooth, W. (1958) Goitre and arteriosclerosis. *Lancet*, **2**, 171
5. Vanhaelst, L., Neve, P., Chailly, P. and Bastenie, P. A. (1967). Coronary-artery disease in hypothyroidism. *Lancet*, **2**, 800
6. Steinberg, A. D. (1968). Myxedema and coronary artery disease – a comparative autopsy study. *Ann. Intern. Med.*, **68**, 338
7. Coronary Drug Project Research Group (1972). The Coronary Drug Project. Findings leading to further modifications of its protocol with respect to dextrothyroxine. *J. Am. Med. Assoc.*, **220**, 996
8. Bastenie, P. A., Vanhaelst, L. and Neve, P. (1967). Coronary-artery disease in hypothyroidism. *Lancet*, **2**, 1221
9. Bastenie, P. A., Vanhaelst, L., Bonnyms, M., Neve, P. and Staquet, M. (1971). Preclinical hypothyroidism: a risk factor for coronary heart disease. *Lancet*, **1**, 203
10. Bastenie, P. A., Vanhaelst, L., Golstein, J. and Smets, P. H. (1977). Asymptomatic autoimmune thyroiditis and coronary heart disease. *Lancet*, **2**, 155
11. Green, W. L., Hazzard, W. R. and Hershman, J. M. (1976). Thyrotropin levels in hyperlipidemic survivors of myocardial infarction. *Metabolism*, **25**, 465
12. Heinonen, O. P., Gordin, A., Aho, K., Punsar, S., Pyorala, K. and Puro, K. (1972). Symptomless autoimmune thyroiditis in coronary heart disease. *Lancet*, **1**, 785
13. Tunbridge, W. M. G., Evered, D. C., Hall, R. *et al.* (1977). Lipid profiles and cardiovascular disease in the Whickham area with particular reference to thyroid failure. *Clin. Endocrinol.*, **7**, 495
14. Tunbridge, W. M. G., Brewis, M., French, J. M. *et al.* (1981). Natural history of autoimmune thyroiditis. *Br. Med. J.*, **282**, 258
15. Fowler, P. B. S. (1977). Premyxoedema – a cause of preventable coronary heart disease. *Proc. R. Soc. Med.*, **70**, 297
16. Gordin, A., Heinonen, O. P., Saarinen, P. and Lamberg, B. A. (1972). Serum-thyrotrophin in symptomless autoimmune thyroiditis. *Lancet*, **1**, 551
17. Whittingham, S., Mathews, J. D., Mackay, I. R., Stocks, A. E., Ungar, B. and Martin, F. I. R. (1971). Diabetes mellitus, autoimmunity and ageing. *Lancet*, **1**, 763
18. Mathews, J. D., Hooper, B. M., Whittingham, S., Mackay, I. R. and Stenhouse, N. S.

(1973). Association of autoantibodies with smoking, cardiovascular morbidity, and death in the Busselton population. *Lancet*, **2,** 754
19. Mathews, J. D., Rodger, B. M. and Stenhouse, N. S. (1976). The significance of the association of tissue autoantibodies and rheumatoid factor with angina in the Busselton population. *J. Chron. Dis.*, **29,** 345
20. Editorial (1977). Thyroiditis, autoimmunity and coronary risk factors. *Lancet*, **2,** 173
21. Barnes, B. O. (1975). Hypertension and the thyroid gland. *Clin. Exp. Pharmacol. Physiol.*, suppl. **2,** 167
22. Hellem, A. J., Segaard, E. and Solem, J. H. (1975). The adhesiveness of human blood platelets and thyroid function. *Acta Med. Scand.*, **197,** 15
23. Nordoy, A., Vik-Mo, H. and Berntsen, H. (1976). Haemostatic and lipid abnormalities in hypothyroidism. *Scand. J. Haematol.*, **16,** 154
24. Nakao, J., Chang, W.-C., Murota, S.-I. and Orimo, H. (1981). Triiodothyronine stimulates prostacyclin production by rat aortic smooth muscle cells in culture. *Atherosclerosis*, **39,** 439
25. Katz-Feigenbaum, D., Braun, L. and Wolinsky, H. (1981). Hydrolase activities in the rat aorta. *Circ. Res.*, **49,** 732
26. Minick, C. R. (1980). Immunologic arterial injury and atherogenesis. In Gotto, A. M., Smith, L. C. and Allen, B. (eds.) *Atherosclerosis*. Vol. V, pp. 330–3. (New York: Springer-Verlag)

15
Thyroid function and lipid metabolism

PLASMA LIPIDS AND LIPOPROTEINS IN THYROID DISORDERS

It has been known for many years that serum cholesterol levels are often elevated in patients with hypothyroidism. Indeed, in earlier years cholesterol was used as an aid to diagnosis in thyroid disease[1,2]. It is only more recently that attention has been paid to the mechanism of the elevation of serum cholesterol in thyroid disease. Much less attention has been paid to serum triglycerides and their relation to thyroid disease is less constant. One of the confounding factors in studies of the relationship of thyroid disease to lipid metabolism is the fact that hyperthyroidism is usually associated with lipid levels within the normal range.

Systematic studies of lipid metabolism in thyroid disease, particularly in hypothyroidism, have been undertaken recently and the pattern of abnormalities has become clearer. Some of the studies have used only small numbers of subjects but the results have been consistent. The more recent studies tend to show that both triglyceride and cholesterol are elevated in myxoedema. Studies of lipoprotein composition suggested that the raised triglyceride was present in very low-density lipoproteins (VLDL). Changes in the fat composition of the diet in hypothyroidism had the same effect on lipid levels as in patients without thyroid disease[3] and treatment with thyroxine reduced both triglyceride and cholesterol levels. In 10 hypothyroid subjects[4] triglyceride levels were raised in nine and after therapy they fell towards the normal range although three still remained abnormal. In seven thyrotoxic subjects fasting plasma triglyceride levels were below or within the normal range and were unchanged by treatment. In another study[5], 69% of hypothyroid patients had raised cholesterol levels, 63% raised triglyceride levels and many subjects had elevation of both lipids. Replacement therapy resulted in significant reductions in plasma cholesterol but smaller and non-significant changes in plasma triglyceride. The authors could not detect differences in individual lipoproteins with treatment. In a different approach to lipid abnormalities in hypothyroidism[6], hypothyroidism was detected in 22 of 1500 patients attending a lipid clinic; 17 had both elevated cholesterol and triglyceride, while treatment with thyroxine produced normal lipid levels in 18 of the 22 subjects.

A number of studies have reported the presence of a lipoprotein of abnormal composition in hypothyroidism. The ratio of cholesterol to triglyceride in VLDL in untreated hypothyroidism was abnormally high compared to that in subjects with normal lipids and normal thyroid function[5]. This is a type of abnormality which is found in type III or broad β-hyperlipoproteinemia and is thought to be due to the accumulation of a remnant or intermediate lipoprotein resulting from partial catabolism of chylomicra. This latter finding is of interest as Hazzard and Bierman[7] reported the aggravation of broad β-disease by hypothyroidism. They studied in detail a man who had extensive atherosclerosis and a history of poorly controlled hypothyroidism. He had the clinical characteristics both of hypothyroidism and of broad β-disease with tuberous and planar xanthomas and the characteristic lipoprotein abnormalities on ultracentrifugation. When his hypothyroidism was effectively treated, his lipid levels returned to normal but the lipoprotein abnormalities, characteristic of broad β-disease, could still be detected. It was suggested that hypothyroidism and a genetically determined abnormality of lipoproteins coexisted in this subject. A high cholesterol to triglyceride ratio in VLDL[8] and a broad β-abnormality on electrophoresis of isolated VLDL[6] have been reported in other studies of hypothyroidism. Substitution therapy reduced the cholesterol to triglyceride ratio.

Two factors which may influence lipid abnormalities in hypothyroidism are obesity and the degree of thyroid deficiency. A study of 10 non-obese and 16 obese hypothyroid subjects found normal triglyceride levels in the former and also in 50% of the latter[9]. Thyroid replacement for only 2 weeks caused a reduction in plasma triglyceride although in some subjects with markedly elevated levels triglycerides did not return to normal. All the hypothyroid subjects had TSH levels greater than 40 mU/l and there was no relationship between TSH and lipid levels. In a group of hyperthyroid subjects triglyceride levels were normal and unchanged by treatment. Another study looked at the effect of substitution treatment in 21 hypothyroid subjects[10] who were divided into two groups by TSH levels below or above 40 mU/l. Serum triglyceride and VLDL levels did not change in either group, but serum cholesterol decreased significantly in the group with severe disease. LDL cholesterol and apoprotein B also decreased in this group. HDL triglyceride decreased in the group with severe disease, HDL cholesterol was unchanged and apoprotein A-I increased slightly. Plasma insulin concentrations increased by 28% in the group with severe disease but glucagon did not change.

It has been suggested that 'premyxoedema', a state in which thyroid function is normal in clinically euthyroid patients, but in which thyroid antibodies or raised serum TSH levels are present, is associated with hypercholesterolaemia[11]. More recent studies in clinic patients[12] and in community surveys[13-15] have failed to confirm these observations. In a detailed study of serum lipids in hypothyroidism[16,] 142 patients with thyroid abnormalities were divided into three groups: euthyroid subjects who had autoimmune thyroiditis or circulating thyroid antibodies, patients with raised TSH responses to TRH, and hypothyroid subjects with low circulating thyroid hormone levels. It was only in the latter group of patients that serum cholesterol was significantly raised. Serum triglycerides were not different from the controls in any of the groups. Serum TSH levels were significantly related to cholesterol but not to triglycerides. On replacement therapy with thyroxine and return to normal of TSH levels there was a significant reduction in the serum cholesterol. Thus patients with autoimmune thyroid disease who were euthyroid and those with mild degrees of thyroid failure had normal serum cholesterol. In this study, no effect of hypothyroidism on serum triglyceride was found.

Two studies have specifically looked at high-density lipoprotein (HDL) levels in thyroid disease and have produced conflicting results. In one study[17] HDL levels were elevated in hypothyroidism and low in hyperthyroidism and returned to normal with treatment of the respective conditions. On the other hand, total and LDL cholesterol were elevated in hypothyroidism and the ratio of total to HDL cholesterol was elevated. In the other study[18] HDL cholesterol levels were lower in both hyperthyroid and hypothyroid subjects than in euthyroid subjects. The explanation for the different results is not clear.

It is difficult to draw firm conclusions on the effect of thyroid disease on lipid levels. The selection of the study subjects, the severity of the thyroid disorder and the presence of other influences on lipid metabolism, including obesity and genetic hyperlipidaemias, may contribute to the varying results in different studies. Hyperthyroidism may result in a slight decrease in lipid and lipoprotein levels but usually not beyond what are generally accepted as normal limits. Hypothyroidism is associated with increased cholesterol levels, and often, particularly when it is severe, with raised triglyceride levels. There is evidence of an association of thyroid deficiency and broad β-lipoproteins. This is of potential importance as this lipoprotein is considered to be particularly atherogenic.

MECHANISM OF LIPID DISORDERS IN HYPOTHYROIDISM

Cholesterol

A number of sophisticated studies of cholesterol metabolism in hypothyroidism have been carried out. One of the earlier studies of mechanisms of alterations of serum lipids in thyroid disease used ^{131}I-labelled low-density lipoproteins (LDL) to study lipoprotein turnover[19]. In thyrotoxicosis, LDL levels were depressed, there was a decrease in LDL pool size and an increased rate of LDL catabolism, with a decreased half-life of LDL. The opposite changes were found in hypothyroidism. Treatment of the thyroid condition with restoration of the euthyroid state was accompanied by a return of these values to normal. In three patients with hypothyroidism the turnover of radioactive-labelled cholesterol was studied before replacement therapy and after administration of thyroxine[20].

The excretion of products of cholesterol metabolism, mainly bile acids and cholesterol, was also studied. The thyroxine-induced fall in the level of serum cholesterol was found to be associated with a marked increase in the excretion of steroids derived from circulating cholesterol. The labelled cholesterol studies also suggested that the synthesis of cholesterol was decreased during replacement treatment. It appears, however, that in hypothyroidism, the major defect in cholesterol metabolism is a decrease in catabolism of cholesterol which is more depressed than cholesterol synthesis resulting in hypercholesterolaemia[21]. Animal experiments have shown similar effects of hypothyroidism on LDL catabolism[22].

Two recent studies have looked at the role of the LDL receptor in the regulation LDL in relation to thyroid hormone activity. In a study[23] of the effect of L-triiodothyronine (T_3) on the binding and degradation of labelled LDL in cultured normal skin fibroblasts it was found that increasing concentrations of T_3 caused an increase in both the binding and degradation of LDL (Figure 15.1). No effects were found in receptor negative cells and kinetic studies indicated that T_3 probably increased LDL receptor number rather than altered the affinity of LDL for its receptor. The effect of T_3 was slow, 24 h being required for the effect to be seen. The relevance of this finding to the *in vivo* regulation of LDL in humans with thyroid disease has been studied by measuring the receptor-mediated

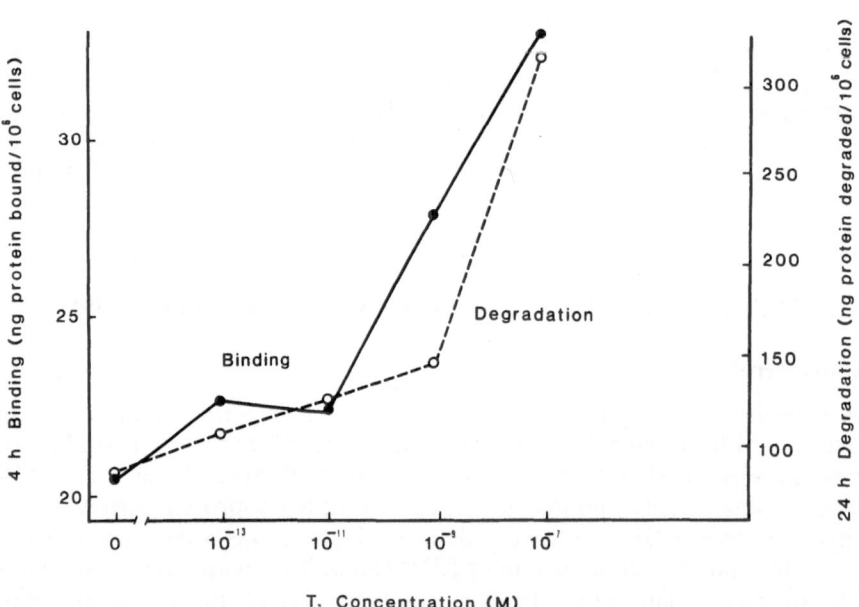

Figure 15.1 Effect of triiodothyronine on LDL binding and degradation in cultured normal human fibroblasts[23]

binding of LDL in a subject with hypothyroidism before and after treatment, using a technique in which the turnover of labelled LDL and labelled LDL which has been treated to inhibit its binding to the receptor were both measured[24]. Before treatment, LDL turnover showed a marked decrease in both receptor-mediated and receptor-independent removal mechanisms. After treatment with thyroxine there were increases in removal, especially through the receptor-mediated pathways. These changes were accompanied by a considerable reduction in LDL concentration.

The overall effect of thyroid hormones on cholesterol and LDL metabolism may be related to their effects on LDL receptor activity. Hence thyroid deficiency results in decreased LDL binding and catabolism, and this is reversed by thyroid replacement. Thyroid hormones also have direct effects on cholesterol synthesis and degradation independent of their effects on the LDL receptor. If LDL receptor activity in arterial cells is regulated by thyroid hormone in the same way as in other cells, receptor-mediated uptake of LDL would seem to be an unlikely mechanism for atherosclerosis in hypothyroidism.

Triglyceride

A number of studies have looked at the mechanism of the raised triglyceride levels in hypothyroidism. Triglyceride levels are a balance between absorption of dietary triglyceride, synthesis of triglyceride in the liver and removal of triglyceride. The latter is mainly related to the activity of the enzyme lipoprotein lipase which exists in two forms: one in adipose tissue and the other in hepatic tissue. Lipoprotein lipase can be indirectly measured by studying the lipolytic activity of plasma after an intravenous injection of heparin – post-heparin lipolytic activity (PHLA). In patients with myxoedema, PHLA levels are low and restored to normal by treatment with thyroxine[25-28]. Triglyceride levels are also restored to normal, suggesting that the two measurements are related in a reciprocal fashion. Lipoprotein lipase has also been measured in adipose tissue biopsies in subjects with hypothyroidism before and after treatment[28]. Lipoprotein lipase was lower in the hypothyroid patients, and with treatment increased to levels comparable with the controls. Changes in PHLA correlated with changes in adipose tissue lipoprotein lipase. There was a significant inverse correlation between plasma triglyceride levels and adipose tissue lipoprotein lipase but no correlation between plasma triglyceride and PHLA. This study suggests again that hypothyroidism is related to low tissue lipoprotein lipase activity and that the activity of this enzyme is dependent on thyroid hormone.

Kinetic studies of triglyceride metabolism in hypothyroidism have been carried out using artificial fat emulsion and native triglycerides. In hypothyroid subjects the clearance of an infused triglyceride load was low before treatment and rose towards normal after treatment with thyroxine[4,8]. In thyrotoxicosis, the triglyceride clearance rates were high or normal and returned towards normal after treatment[4]. Plasma endogenous triglyceride transport kinetics have been determined in 16 hyperthyroid and 12 hypothyroid subjects[27]. In thyrotoxicosis, triglyceride levels were slightly increased above those of control subjects. This was associated with an augmented production of triglyceride but no change in fractional removal rate. Removal of exogenous lipid and PHLA were also above normal in thyrotoxicosis. In hypothyroidism, the synthesis of plasma triglycerides was normal but the fractional removal both of endogenous and exogenous triglyceride was markedly reduced. This was accompained by a decrease in PHLA. Plasma free fatty acid (FFA) and glycerol levels were increased in hyperthyroidism and FFA slightly decreased in hypothyroidism, but these were not correlated with any measurement of triglyceride metabolism.

In another study of plasma triglycerides in hypothyroidism and hyperthyroidism in man[9] it was found that hypothyroidism itself, especially in the absence of obesity, rarely induced clinical hypertriglyceridaemia. On the other hand, about half the obese patients had elevated plasma triglycerides and in a few cases the increases were marked. The treatment of hypothyroid patients generally caused a reduction in plasma triglyceride. Thus the hypothyroid state apparently caused a slight increase in triglyceride but usually not to abnormally high levels. However, most of those with striking elevations of triglyceride did not normalize their lipids after treatment, suggesting that they had an underlying primary hypertriglyceridaemia perhaps accentuated by obesity. Patients with hyperthyroidism almost always had normal plasma triglycerides in the untreated state and the values were essentially unchanged by therapy. PHLA was normal in hypothyroidism and not changed by treatment. In contrast, hepatic triglyceride lipase (HTGL) was reduced in hypothyroidism and increased with thyroid replacement. HTGL was slightly higher than normal in patients with hyperthyroidism. Thyroid disease itself did not appear to have consistent effects on chylomicron clearance and the majority of patients with hypothyroidism who had normal triglyceride levels, had normal fractional clearance rates of VLDL. Although before treatment, obese hypothyroid subjects had an excess production of VLDL they also had a relative defect in clearance of VLDL. This was reversed by thyroid hormone replacement. Thus, triglyceride metabolism is not grossly deranged in hypothyroidism but thyroid hormones can promote catabolism of VLDL.

Thyroid hormones influence both the production and removal of plasma triglyceride in man. In hyperthyroidism the mean alteration is increased synthesis of endogenous plasma triglyceride. In hypothyroidism impaired removal of triglyceride occurs, related to a decrease in the activity of lipoprotein lipase, the enzyme mainly responsible for catabolism of this lipid.

CONCLUSIONS

Thyroid deficiency tends to cause elevations of both triglyceride and cholesterol levels. This is related to impairment in removal mechanisms mediated respectively by lipoprotein lipase and the LDL receptor mechanism. An abnormal cholesterol-rich VLDL may occur in hypothyroidism. Hyperthyroidism tends to cause reductions in both lipid levels but the changes are small. The effects of thyroid disorders on lipid metabolism are influenced by the severity of the disorder and modified by coexisting obesity or genetic hyperlipoproteinaemias.

References

1. Peters, J. P. and Man, E. B. (1950). The significance of serum cholesterol in thyroid disease. *J. Clin. Invest.*, **29**, 1
2. Malmros, H. and Swahn, B. (1953). Lipid metabolism in myxedema. *Acta Med. Scand.*, **145**, 361
3. O'Hara, D. D., Porte, D., Jr and Williams, R. H. (1966). The effect of diet and thyroxin on plasma lipids in myxedema. *Metabolism*, **15**, 123
4. Tulloch, B. R., Lewis, B. and Fraser, T. R. (1973). Triglyceride metabolism in thyroid disease. *Lancet*, **1**, 391
5. Wahlqvist, M. L., Fidge, N. H. and Lomas, F. (1977). Lipoprotein composition in hypothyroidism. *Clin. Chim. Acta*, **77**, 269
6. Mishkel, M. A. and Crowther, S. M. (1977). Hypothyroidism, an important cause of reversible hyperlipidemia. *Clin. Chim. Acta*, **74**, 139
7. Hazzard, W. R. and Bierman, E. L. (1972). Aggravation of broad β disease (type 3 hyperlipoproteinemia) by hypothyroidism. *Arch. Intern. Med.*, **130**, 822
8. Rossner, S. and Rosenqvist, U. (1974). Serum lipoproteins and the intravenous fat tolerance test in hypothyroid patients before and during substitution therapy. *Atherosclerosis*, **20**, 365
9. Abrams, J. J., Grundy, S. M. and Ginsberg, H. (1981). Metabolism of plasma triglycerides in hypothyroidism and hyperthyroidism in man. *J. Lipid Res.*, **22**, 307
10. Lithell, H., Boberg, J., Hellsing, K. *et al.* (1981). Serum lipoprotein and apolipoprotein concentrations and tissue lipoprotein–lipase activity in overt and subclinical hypothyroidism: the effect of substitution therapy. *Eur. J. Clin. Invest.*, **11**, 3
11. Fowler, P. B. S., Swale, J. and Andrews, H. (1970). Hypercholesterolaemia in borderline hypothyroidism stage of premyxoedema. *Lancet*, **2**, 488
12. Nilsson, G., Nordlander, S. and Levin, K. (1976). Studies on subclinical hypothyroidism with special reference to the serum lipid pattern. *Acta Med. Scand.*, **200**, 63
13. Green, W. L., Hazzard, W. R. and Hershman, J. M. (1976). Thyrotropin levels in hyperlipidemic survivors of myocardial infarction. *Metabolism*, **25**, 465
14. Tunbridge, W. M. G., Evered, D. C., Hall, R. *et al.* (1977). Lipid profiles and cardiovascular disease in the Whickham area with particular reference to thyroid failure. *Clin. Endocrinol.*, **7**, 495
15. Tunbridge, W. M. G., Brewis, M., French, J. M. *et al.* (1981). Natural history of autoimmune thyroiditis. *Br. Med. J.*, **282**, 258
16. Kutty, K. M., Bryant, D. G. and Farid, N. R. (1978). Serum lipids in hypothyroidism – a re-evaluation. *J. Clin. Endocrinol. Metab.*, **46**, 55
17. Scottolini, A. G., Bhagavan, N. V., Oshiro, T. H. and Abe, S. Y. (1980). Serum high-density lipoprotein cholesterol concentrations in hypo- and hyperthyroidism. *Clin. Chem.*, **26**, 584
18. Agdeppa, D., Macaron, C., Mallik, T. and Schnuda, N. D. (1979). Plasma high density lipoprotein cholesterol in thyroid disease. *J. Clin. Endocrinol. Metab.*, **49**, 726
19. Walton, K. W., Scott, P. J., Dykes, P. W. and Davies, J. W. L. (1965). The significance of alterations in serum lipids in thyroid dysfunction. *Clin. Sci.*, **29**, 217
20. Miettinen, T. A. (1968). Mechanism of serum cholesterol reduction by thyroid hormones in hypothyroidism. *J. Lab. Clin. Med.*, **71**, 537
21. Abrams, J. J. and Grundy, S. M. (1981). Cholesterol metabolism in hypothyroidism and hyperthyroidism in man. *J. Lipid Res.*, **22**, 323
22. Sykes, M., Cnoop-Koopmans, W. M., Julien, P. and Angel, A. (1981). The effects of

hypothyroidism, age and nutrition on LDL catabolism in the rat. *Metabolism*, **30**, 733

23. Chait, A., Bierman, E. L. and Albers, J. J. (1979). Regulatory role of triiodothyronine in the degradation of low density lipoprotein by cultured human skin fibroblasts. *J. Clin. Endocrinol. Metab.*, **48**, 887

24. Thompson, G. R., Soutar, A. K., Spengel, F. A., Jadhav, A., Gavigan, S. J. P. and Myant, N. B. (1981). Defects of receptor-mediated low density lipoprotein catabolism in homozygous familial hypercholesterolemia and hypothyroidism in vivo. *Proc. Natl. Acad. Sci., USA*, **78**, 2591

25. Porte, D., Jr, O'Hara, D. D. and Williams, R. H. (1966). The relation between postheparin lipolytic activity and plasma triglyceride in myxedema. *Metabolism*, **15**, 107

26. Kirkeby, K. (1968). Postheparin plasma lipoprotein lipase activity in thyroid disease. *Acta Endocrinol.*, **59**, 555

27. Nikkila, E. A. and Kekki, M. (1972). Plasma triglyceride metabolism in thyroid disease. *J. Clin. Invest.*, **51**, 2103

28. Pykalisto, O., Goldberg, A. P. and Brunzell, J. D. (1976). Reversal of decreased human adipose tissue lipoprotein lipase and hypertriglyceridemia after treatment of hypothyroidism. *J. Clin. Endocrinol. Metab.*, **43**, 591

OTHER HORMONES

16
Growth hormone

GROWTH HORMONE AND CARDIOVASCULAR DISEASE

Acromegaly is associated with a high frequency of cardiac disease[1]. Cardiac enlargement is the most characteristic abnormality, but hypertension and cardiac failure also occur.

Acromegaly is an uncommon disease and detailed studies of the cardiovascular system in large series of acromegalic subjects have been rare. A prospective study of 57 patients with acromegaly found clinical evidence of coronary heart disease in two[2]. Eight patients died, and at autopsy one had severe coronary atherosclerosis and two had mild to moderate coronary disease. Hypertension, usually mild, was the commonest cardiovascular abnormality. The findings of a detailed clinical and pathological study of 27 cases of acromegaly presenting to the Mayo Clinic over a 60-year period have recently been published[3]. Cardiac hypertrophy and hypertension were common but not related. However, significant coronary atherosclerosis was less common, being found in 11%, and old myocardial infarction in 15%. Significant aortic atherosclerosis was found in 24%. Most of the patients with significant atherosclerosis were in the older age groups. 15% of acromegaly subjects were diabetic. These studies do not support the view that premature or accelerated atherosclerosis occurs in acromegaly.

Further evidence of a possible association of growth hormone and atherosclerosis comes from studies on patients with isolated growth hormone deficiency. Growth hormone-deficient dwarfs have abnormal glucose tolerance, variable insulin secretion, and about 50% have elevated cholesterol or triglyceride levels[4]. Despite this, only two of 31 dwarfs had clinical or ECG evidence of atherosclerotic heart disease. A later follow-up study[5] confirmed that despite hyperglycaemia and hyperlipidaemia the prevalence of clinical atherosclerosis was much lower than in age- and sex-matched diabetics. While this suggests that growth hormone may be necessary for the development of atherosclerosis, the very low insulin levels in the growth hormone-deficient dwarfs may also be significant.

GROWTH HORMONE AND LIPID METABOLISM

Studies of serum lipids in acromegaly have produced conflicting results. In the largest and most detailed study lipid metabolism was investigated in 46 patients with active acromegaly[6]. The mean serum cholesterol was lower in the acromegalic subjects than in normal controls. Mean serum triglyceride was increased in the acromegalics, hypertriglyceridaemia being present in 32% of males and 19% of females. Nine acromegalic patients had diabetes, but the high prevalence of diabetes did not account for the raised triglyceride levels, nor did serum triglyceride correlate with body weight. Serum cholesterol and triglyceride levels did not correlate with growth hormone levels. However, acromegalic patients with higher serum insulin levels had higher serum triglycerides than those with lower insulin levels. Treatment of the acromegaly returned lipid and carbohydrate metabolism towards normal. A low frequency of hyperlipidaemia was reported in another group of 24 acromegalic subjects[7] but the study included patients who had been treated and those who had low growth hormone levels.

Possible mechanisms for hypertriglyceridaemia in acromegaly include decreased lipoprotein lipase and hepatic triglyceride lipase[8] and increased triglyceride synthesis[9] under the influence of high insulin levels[10].

Growth hormone deficiency is associated with raised plasma cholesterol and triglyceride levels[4,5]. However this may be because growth hormone deficiency unmasks an underlying abnormality in lipoprotein metabolism, rather than causing hyperlipidaemia[11].

The relationship of growth hormone to individual lipoproteins is not clear. In hypopituitarism, total cholesterol and triglyceride were slightly increased and HDL was decreased[12]. However, HDL levels returned to normal on therapy with thyroid hormone and prednisone. In one subject with isolated growth hormone deficiency HDL was decreased, but in three subjects with acromegaly, HDL was normal or low.

The role of growth hormone in the regulation of lipid and lipoprotein metabolism remains unclear. There is no consistent evidence that acromegaly is associated with lipid abnormalities that would predispose to atherosclerosis.

GROWTH HORMONE AND EXPERIMENTAL ATHEROSCLEROSIS

There has been very little reported work on the relation of growth hormone levels to experimental atherosclerosis and the biology of the arterial wall. Growth hormone deficiency can be produced by hypophysectomy but this also produces changes in the secretion of other hormones. Replacement treatment with growth hormone may help to identify its effects, but there is such close interaction among hormones that even this may be uninformative.

Hypophysectomy in dogs causes changes in aortic connective tissue. Elastin and DNA were increased but glycosaminoglycan concentrations were reduced[13]. Growth hormone administration resulted in return towards normal in elastin, dermatan sulphate and chondroitin sulphate. However, although hypophysectomy resulted in similar effects on the coronary arteries, growth hormone had no effect[14]. It was concluded that there is a differential sensitivity to growth hormone of different parts of the arterial system.

Serum from human diabetics[15] or from animals with experimental diabetes[16] stimulates the growth of rabbit aortic smooth muscle cells in primary culture. This process is inhibited by growth hormone antiserum[17] and growth of arterial smooth muscle cells is stimulated by growth hormone[18]. Growth hormone also stimulates connective tissue formation in cultured rabbit aortic smooth muscle cells[19].

The finding of a direct effect of growth hormone on proliferation of aortic smooth muscle cells is surprising as growth hormone is thought not to act directly on tissues but by way of other growth factors or somatomedins. Somatomedins A and C stimulate growth of cultured rat aortic smooth muscle cells[20]. It is possible that growth hormone added to medium containing serum acted indirectly by way of another growth factor.

The rather scanty evidence available suggests that growth hormone may have a role in the regulation of aortic connective tissue. However, there is doubt as to whether growth hormone itself has potent biological effects or whether it acts through an intermediate substance. In any case the relevance of the effects to the pathogenesis of atherosclerosis is not clear.

CONCLUSIONS

The case for an association between growth hormone secretion and atherosclerosis is unimpressive. There is little good evidence that acromegaly is associated with accelerated atherosclerosis, and the lack of vascular disease in growth hormone-deficient dwarfs may be due to factors other than low circulating growth hormone levels. Growth hormone does not appear to have effects on lipid metabolism or on the arterial wall that would predispose to atherosclerosis.

References

1. Wright, A. D., Hill, D. M., Lowy, C. and Fraser, T. R. (1970). Mortality in acromegaly. *Q. J. Med.*, **39**, 1
2. McGuffin, W. L., Sherman, B. M., Roth, J. *et al.* (1974). Acromegaly and cardiovascular disorders. *Ann. Intern. Med.*, **81**, 11
3. Lie, J. T. and Grossman, S. J. (1980). Pathology of the heart in acromegaly: anatomic findings in 27 autopsied patients. *Am. Heart J.*, **100**, 41
4. Merimee, T. J., Fineberg, S. E. and Hollander, W. (1973). Vascular disease in the chronic HDH-deficient state. *Diabetes*, **22**, 813
5. Merimee, T. J. (1978). A follow-up study of vascular disease in growth-hormone-deficient dwarfs with diabetes. *N. Engl. J. Med.*, **298**, 1217
6. Nikkila, E. A. and Pelkonen, R. (1975). Serum lipids in acromegaly. *Metabolism*, **24**, 829
7. Aloia, J. F., Roginsky, M. S. and Field, R. A. (1972). Absence of hyperlipidemia in acromegaly. *J. Clin. Endocrinol. Metab.*, **35**, 921

8. Murase, T., Yamada, N., Ohsawa, N., Kosaka, K., Morita, S. and Yoshida, S. (1980). Decline of postheparin plasma lipoprotein lipase in acromegalic patients. *Metabolism*, **29**, 666

9. Friedman, M., Byers, S. O., Rosenman, R. H., Li, C. H. and Newman, R. (1974). Effect of subacute administration of human growth hormone on various serum lipid and hormone levels of hypercholesterolemic and normocholesterolemic subjects. *Metabolism*, **23**, 905

10. Trimble, E. R., Atkinson, A. B., Buchanan, K. D. and Hadden, D. R. (1980). Plasma glucagon and insulin concentrations in acromegaly. *J. Clin. Endocrinol. Metab.*, **51**, 626

11. Merimee, T. J. (1980). Familial combined hyperlipoproteinemia. Evidence for a role of growth hormone deficiency in effecting its manifestation. *J. Clin. Invest.*, **65**, 829

12. Sagel, J., Lopes-Virella, M. F., Levine, J. H. and Colwell, J. A. (1979). Decreased high density lipoprotein cholesterol in hypopituitarism. *J. Clin. Endocrinol. Metab.*, **49**, 753

13. Brosnan, M. E., Sirek, O. V., Sirek, A. and Przybylska, K. (1973). Action of growth hormone and thyroxine on aortas of hypophysectomised dogs. *Diabetes*, **22**, 243

14. Sirek, O. V., Sirek, A., Fikar, K. and Przybylska, K. (1976). Lack of somatotropin effect on glycosaminoglycan content of canine coronary arteries. *Endocrinology*, **99**, 1448

15. Ledet, T. (1976). Growth of rabbit aortic smooth muscle cells in serum from patients with juvenile diabetes. *Acta Pathol. Microbiol. Scand, Sect. A.*, **84**, 508

16. Ledet, T., Fischer-Dzoga, K. and Wissler, R. W. (1976). Growth of rabbit aortic smooth-muscle cells cultured in media containing diabetic and hyperlipemic serum. *Diabetes*, **25**, 207

17. Ledet, T. (1977). Growth hormone antiserum suppresses the growth effect of diabetic serum. *Diabetes*, **26**, 798

18. Ledet, T. (1976). Growth hormone stimulates the growth of arterial medial cells *in vitro*. *Diabetes*, **25**, 1011

19. Ledet, T. and Luust, J. (1980). Arterial procollagen type I, type III and fibronectin. Effects of diabetic serum, glucose, insulin, ketones and growth hormone studied on rabbit aortic myomedial cell cultures. *Diabetes*, **29**, 964

20. Weinstein, R., Stemerman, M. B. and Maciag, T. (1981). Hormonal requirements for growth of arterial smooth muscle cells *in vitro*: an endocrine approach to atherosclerosis. *Science*, **212**, 818

17
Renin

HYPERTENSION AND ATHEROSCLEROSIS

Hypertension is one of the major risk factors for atherosclerosis[1]. Stroke and congestive cardiac failure are the most important complications of raised blood pressure (Table 17.1) but myocardial infarction also has a close association with hypertension. There is good evidence from a number of well-designed trials[3,4] that therapeutic reduction of raised blood pressure prevents many of the complications of hypertension (Table 17.2).

Table 17.1 Risk of cardiovascular disease in 14 years in men aged 30–62 years with normal or high blood pressure

	Blood pressure	
	Normal	High
Coronary heart disease	70	133
Intermittent claudication	67	140
Stroke	51	184
Congestive heart failure	54	237

Normal blood pressure is a pressure of 140/90 mmHg or less, and high blood pressure 160/95 mmHg or more. The figures represent the ratio of observed to expected cases (Framingham study[2])

Blood pressure is related to vascular disease in a number of different ways, not all of which are associated with atherosclerosis[5]. The mechanical effects of prolonged exposure to high blood pressure cause myocardial hypertrophy and predispose to cardiac failure. Myocardial ischaemia augments this process. The direct mechanical effects of high blood pressure may also contribute to aneurysm formation in both the aorta and the cerebral arteries. Extreme elevation of blood pressure (malignant hypertension) is associated with necrosis of blood vessels, particularly

Table 17.2 Effect of treatment of hypertension on some fatal and non-fatal complications (Veterans Administration study[4])

	Control	Treated
Deaths		
Cerebrovascular	7	1
Myocardial infarction	3	2
Aneurysm	1	1
Sudden	8	4
TOTALS	19	8
Non-fatal events		
Cerebrovascular	5	0
Cardiac failure	5	0
Dissecting aortic aneurysm	1	0
Others	5	1
TOTALS	16	1

arterioles. Prolonged hypertension of lesser severity is associated with atherosclerosis.

Most of the studies relating blood pressure to cardiovascular disease have been clinical and epidemiological. They have suffered not only from possible lack of precision in the diagnosis of cardiovascular disease but also from problems in measuring blood pressure and in defining hypertension. The best investigation is the Framingham prospective study[1] which has identified a relationship between blood pressure and congestive cardiac failure, myocardial infarction, stroke and intermittent claudication (Table 17.1). The risk is progressive with rising blood pressure, is associated with both systolic and diastolic arterial pressure, and starts at pressures which are within what is usually regarded as the normal range. Studies of this type do not identify the nature of the vascular disease but the fact that hypertension is associated with such widespread arterial disease suggests that atherosclerosis is at least partly responsible.

Post-mortem studies of arterial disease in relation to blood pressure are also difficult to interpret. Blood pressure may have been measured ante-mortem but this may have been during a terminal illness, which may itself have affected blood pressure. Blood pressures in clinical records have not usually been measured by standardized techniques. An alternative to using clinical records is to diagnose hypertension on the basis of post-mortem evidence of other complications of high blood pressure. Left ventricular hypertrophy in the absence of valvular disease is often used as evidence of hypertension. However, this definition lacks precision. In the International Atherosclerosis Project[6] hypertension was defined by clinical or pathological criteria. Hypertension was associated with an increase in fatty streaks in both the aorta and coronary arteries, and in raised atherosclerotic lesions. The prevalence of fibrous plaques, complicated lesions, calcified lesions and coronary artery stenoses was higher in the hypertensive subjects. Although the diagnosis of hypertension was imprecise, the study provides convincing evidence that hypertension accelerates atherosclerosis.

RENIN AND CARDIOVASCULAR DISEASE

The mechanism by which hypertension predisposes to atherosclerosis is unknown. A deleterious mechanical effect of high pressure on the arterial wall has been suggested, but a mechanism by which this effect causes atherosclerosis has not been described. Damage to the endothelium analogous to the necrotic changes found in arterioles in accelerated hypertension is another possible mechanism but is also speculative[5].

In the last decade there has been controversy about a suggested endocrine mechanism for the cardiovascular complications of hypertension. Hypertension may be associated with changes in the renin–angiotensin–aldosterone system[7,8]. This endocrine system, which is chiefly concerned with regulation of sodium metabolism, is activated by the secretion of renin from the juxtaglomerular apparatus of the kidney. Renin acts on a circulating polypeptide, angiotensinogen, to produce angiotensin I, II, and III. Angiotensin II is the active product and it in turn stimulates secretion of aldosterone from the adrenal cortex. Aldosterone acts on the distal convoluted tubule of the nephron causing sodium retention and potassium excretion.

It has been suggested that when renin levels are related to urinary sodium excretion, hypertensives can be divided into those with low, normal or high renin secretion[9]. Those with high renin levels include patients with severe and accelerated hypertension. It was also suggested that renin secretion correlates with the cardiovascular complications of hypertension and that low renin hypertension is not associated with cardiovascular disease. Later studies have, with one exception, not supported the idea that low renin hypertension does not predispose to cardiovascular disease (Table 17.3).

This suggestion has aroused a considerable amount of controversy since it was first published[16-18]. The protagonists have produced further evidence to support the hypothesis while other investigations have published results which contradict the original proposition. Each side criticizes the other's techniques. The controversy cannot be resolved at present, and will not be resolved until standard methods of measuring renin secretion are available. When this happens, prospective studies will be needed to test the hypothesis.

Brunner and his colleagues suggested that low renin hypertension may not require treatment, and that some methods of treating hypertension might be harmful as they tend to raise plasma renin levels[9]. Nevertheless, the Veterans Administration trials on the treatment of hypertension used thiazide diuretics to lower blood pressure[3,4]. Despite the fact that these

Table 17.3 Results of some studies relating cardiovascular disease (stroke and myocardial infarction) in hypertensive subjects to plasma renin levels (percentages)

	Renin		
	Low	Middle	High
Brunner et al., 1972[9]	0	11	14
Christlieb et al., 1974[10]	0	24	33
Mroczek et al., 1973[11]	10	9	9
Stroobandt et al., 1973[12]	20	21	25
Genest et al., 1973[13]	24	20	45
Doyle ee al., 1973[14]	27	32	17
Gulati et al., 1973 [15]	15	5	–

drugs tend to raise plasma renin levels, their use in hypertension resulted in a reduction in cardiovascular disease.

RENIN AND EXPERIMENTAL ATHEROSCLEROSIS

Although the acute effect of renin and other hormones and enzymes involved in the pathogenesis of hypertension, such as vasopressin, catecholamines and angiotensin II, has been studied on arterial wall structure and metabolism[5], only one group has investigated the effect of changes in renin secretion on experimental atherosclerosis. In one series of experiments, normal and cholesterol-fed rabbits were made hypertensive by placing a clip on one renal artery[19]. The clipped animals were subdivided 3 months later into those with high and those with normal plasma renin activity. As expected, aortic lesions were more common in the cholesterol-fed animals. Hypertension also accelerated aortic lesion formation in the cholesterol-fed animals. However, elevated renin had neither an independent nor a synergistic effect on aortic lesions (Table 17.4). In a second series of experiments renin was depressed by adding saline to the drinking water and injecting 11-desoxycorticosterone (DOC) in normal and cholesterol-fed rabbits[20]. This treatment had no effect on arterial pressure. As before, aortic lesions only occurred in the cholesterol-fed animals, but there was no difference between the normal renin animals and the low renin animals (Table 17.5). Thus, in this experimental model, elevated renin levels did not accelerate atherosclerosis nor did a low-renin state protect against lesion formation. The suggestion that renin secretion has pathological significance in the cardiovascular complications of hypertension remains without experimental support.

Table 17.4 Aortic lesions in relation to plasma renin activity in normal and cholesterol-fed rabbits with unilateral renal artery clips (percentages).

	Normal diet		High-cholesterol diet	
	Normal renin	High renin	Normal renin	High renin
No of animals with lesions	44	86	100	100
Surface area involved by lesions	2.6±3.8	3.1±3.1	64±21	67±30

None of the differences between the normal and high renin groups are significant (Overturf et al.[19])

Table 17.5 Aortic lesions in relation to plasma renin in rabbits fed a normal and high cholesterol diet (percentages)

	Normal diet		High-cholesterol diet	
	Normal renin	Low renin	Normal renin	Low renin
No. of animals with lesions	0	0	100	100
Surface area of lesions	0	0	40±23	50±23

None of the differences between the normal and low renin groups are significant (Overturf et al.[20])

CONCLUSIONS

The hypothesis that plasma renin is a determinant of the development of heart attack and stroke in hypertension remains unproven. Standardized methodology and well-controlled prospective studies are needed to confirm an association between plasma renin and cardiovascular disease. Experimental evidence from animal models of atherosclerosis, or from studies of isolated arteries or arterial cells, is also needed. It is difficult to disagree with the view that 'both the protagonists and antagonists . . . have tended to grossly underestimate the epidemiological problems involved in evaluating a situation containing so many potential variables'[21].

186   HORMONES AND ATHEROSCLEROSIS

References

1. Kannel, W. B. and Dawber, T. R. (1974). Hypertension as an ingredient of a cardiovascular risk profile. *Br. J. Hosp. Med.*, **11**, 508
2. Kannel, W. B., Wolf, P. A., Verter, J. and McNamara, P. M. (1970). Epidemiologic assessment of the role of blood pressure in stroke. The Framingham study. *J. Am. Med. Assoc.*, **214**, 301
3. Veterans Administration Co-operative Study Group on Antihypertensive Agents (1967). Effects of treatment on morbidity in hypertension. Results in patients with diastolic blood pressures averaging 115 through 129 mmHg. *J. Am. Med. Assoc.*, **202**, 1028
4. Veterans Administration Co-operative Study Group on Antihypertensive Agents (1970). Effects of treatment on morbidity in hypertension. II. Results in patients with diastolic blood pressure averaging 90 through 114 mmHg. *J. Am. Med. Assoc.*, **213**, 1143
5. Giese, J. (1973). Renin, angiotensin and hypertensive vascular damage: a review. *Am. J. Med.*, **55**, 315
6. Robertson, W. B. and Strong, J. P. (1968). Atherosclerosis in persons with hypertension and diabetes mellitus. *Lab. Invest.*, **18**, 538
7. Editorial (1972). Angiotensin, myocardial infarction and strokes. *Lancet*, **1**, 1273
8. Laragh, J. H. (1978). The renin system in high blood pressure, from disbelief to reality: converting-enzyme blockade for analysis and treatment. *Prog. Cardiovasc. Dis.*, **21**, 159
9. Brunner, H. R., Laragh, J. H., Baer, L. *et al.* (1972) Essential hypertension: renin and aldosterone, heart attack and stroke. *N. Engl. J. Med.*, **286**, 441
10. Christlieb, A. R., Gleason, R. E., Hickler, R. B. and Lauler, D. P. (1974). Renin: a risk factor for cardiovascular disease? *Ann. Intern. Med.*, **81**, 7
11. Mroczek, W. J., Finnerty, F. A. and Catt, K. J. (1973). Lack of association between plasma-renin and history of heart-attack or stroke in patients with essential hypertension. *Lancet*, **2**, 464
12. Stroobandt, R., Fagard, R. and Amery, A. K. P. C. (1973). Are patients with essential hypertension and low renin protected against stroke and heart attack? *Am. Heart J.*, **86**, 781
13. Genest, J., Boucher, R., Kuchel, O. and Nowaczynski, W. (1973). Renin in hypertension: how important as a risk factor? *Can. Med. Assoc. J.*, **109**, 475
14. Doyle, A. E., Jerums, G., Johnston, C. I. and Louis, W. J. (1973). Plasma renin levels and vascular complications. *Br. Med. J.*, **2**, 206
15. Gulati, S. C., Adlin, V., Biddle, C. M., Marks, A. D. and Channick, B. J. (1973). The occurrence of vascular complications in low renin hypertension. *Ann. Intern. Med.*, **78**, 828
16. Kaplan, N. M. (1975). The prognostic implications of plasma renin in essential hypertension. *J. Am. Med. Assoc.*, **231**, 167
17. Kirkendall, W. M., Hammond, J. J. and Overturf, M. L. (1978). Renin as a predictor of hypertensive complications. *Ann. NY Acad. Sci.*, **304**, 147
18. Laragh, J. H. (1978). Renin as a predictor of hypertensive complications – discussion. *Ann. NY Acad. Sci.*, **304**, 165
19. Overturf, M. L., Aschenbrener, C., Druilhet, R. E. and Kirkendall, W. M. (1981). Renin as a risk factor for atherogenesis. *Atherosclerosis*, **38**, 97
20. Overturf, M. L., Sybers, H. D., Druilhet, R. E. and Kirkendall, W. M. (1981). Renin as a risk factor for atherogenesis. *Atherosclerosis*, **40**, 203
21. Beevers, D. G., Brown, J. J., Fraser, R. *et al.* (1975). The clinical value of renin and angiotensin estimations. *Kidney Int.*, **8**, S181

18
Corticosteriods

CORTICOSTEROIDS AND CLINICAL ATHEROSCLEROSIS

There has been only one study relating circulating corticosteroid hormone levels to clinical atherosclerosis[1]. Seventy-one men had coronary angiography and serum cortisol levels measured during an oral glucose load. There were significant correlations between elevated serum cortisol levels and moderate to severe coronary atherosclerosis. Plasma cortisol was also associated with several risk factors for atherosclerosis, including cholesterol, blood pressure and smoking.

Less direct evidence of an association between corticosteroids and atherosclerosis has come from an autopsy study of 36 patients with systemic lupus erythematosus[2]. Extramural coronary artery narrowing of more than 50% was found in 25% of the subjects and intramural coronary artery narrowing in 56%. Eight of the nine subjects with extramural coronary artery narrowing, and 12 of the 20 subjects with intramural coronary artery narrowing, had been on steroids for more than 12 months. In contrast, a study of similar patients carried out before steroids became available revealed no coronary artery narrowing. Accelerated atherosclerosis also occurs in patients with chronic renal failure treated with dialysis[3] or transplantation[4]. Corticosteroid therapy is often used in this condition, particularly in the prevention of transplant rejection. Patients with rheumatoid arthritis who had been treated with corticosteroids for more than 6 months, had three times as great a prevalence of calcified lesions in the tibial arteries as patients not taking steroids[5]. However the lesions consisted of calcification of the media and were not characteristic of atherosclerosis. Excess lipid deposition in the aorta has also been reported in children receiving cortisone or ACTH as treatment for leukaemia[6].

A review of seven autopsied cases of Cushing's syndrome, together with 107 post-mortem examinations reported in the literature, found that cardiovascular disease was the cause of death in 40%[7]. Cardiac failure was the commonest cardiovascular cause of death. Accelerated atherosclerosis was also found in a later series of 50 patients with Cushing's syndrome[8]. However, 88% of the patients had hypertension and 84% had abnormal glucose tolerance. Both of these may predispose to atherosclerosis.

The clinical situations quoted are complex and it would be unjustifiable to try to isolate any one factor as a cause of cardiovascular disease. Nevertheless, the evidence suggests that high concentrations of corticosteroids may be associated with cardiovascular disease.

A recent review has concluded that 'anxiety, depression, insomnia and "type A behaviour" are consistently related to the risk of coronary disease'[9]. Type A behaviour is characterized by competitiveness, impatience, time consciousness, intense driving for achievement and an excess of drive and hostility. Prospective studies have shown that people with 'type A behaviour' have a higher incidence of coronary artery disease than those with the more placid 'type B behaviour'[10]. Although coronary artery disease was also associated with other risk factors including hyperlipidaemia, hypertension, diabetes and smoking, the association of type A behaviour with coronary artery disease was independent of these factors. Type A behaviour is associated with raised plasma ACTH but normal plasma cortisol levels[11], suggesting that the adrenal is relatively resistant to stimulation. Type A behaviour is also associated with raised plasma cholesterol levels.

LIPID AND CARBOHYDRATE METABOLISM

Corticosteroid treatment may have marked effects on lipid and carbohydrate metabolism. For example, in two patients receiving high-dose prednisone therapy[12], plasma triglyceride levels correlated closely with the prednisone dose. The elevated triglyceride levels were associated with reduced levels of lipoprotein lipase, measured as post-heparin lipolytic activity. High-dose prednisone was also associated with fasting hyperglycaemia, abnormal glucose tolerance and decreased insulin secretion. This contrasts with the more frequent association of steroid therapy with glucose intolerance and elevated insulin secretion, due to resistance to insulin's action[13].

EXPERIMENTAL ATHEROSCLEROSIS

Studies of the effects of corticosteroids on experimental atherosclerosis have produced different results in different species. Thus, hydrocortisone and ACTH had no effect on cholesterol-induced lesions in cockerels despite causing increased lipid and glucose levels, but cortisone increased arterial lesions[14]. In cholesterol-fed rabbits, cortisone inhibited the development of atheromatous lesions without lowering plasma cholesterol levels[15]. The effect on the aorta seemed to be inhibition of cellular proliferation without a reduction in cholesterol uptake. Cortisone also decreased the frequency of spontaneous fibrous plaques in chickens[16]. However, hydrocortisone had little effect on spontaneous lesions in chickens[17]. ACTH increased serum cholesterol levels and aortic lesions in cholesterol-fed hypothyroid dogs[18].

In cultured human aortic smooth muscle cells, serum from patients taking corticosteroid treatment stimulated cell proliferation[19] while in a serum-free medium, hydrocortisone stimulated proliferation of rat aortic smooth muscle cells[20]. However cortisol decreased the synthesis of the glycosaminoglycan, hyaluronic acid by cultured human aortic smooth muscle cells[21,22].

The effect of corticosteroids on lipid metabolism in cultured arterial cells does not appear to have been studied. However, in cultured human skin fibroblasts, physiological concentrations of hydrocortisone decreased LDL uptake and degradation without affecting binding, and reduced sterol synthesis[23].

CONCLUSIONS

The evidence linking abnormal corticosteroid levels with atherosclerosis is weak and the possibility that the association is indirect has not been excluded. The data are not persuasive enough to suggest that a large prospective epidemiological study would be worthwhile. The experimental evidence is not consistent with corticosteroids directly promoting the development of atherosclerosis. It is possible that an association between corticosteroids and atherosclerosis is mediated by changes in carbohydrate metabolism and insulin secretion.

References

1. Troxler, R. G., Sprague, E. A., Albanese, R. A., Fuchs, R. and Thompson, A. J. (1977). The association of elevated plasma cortisol and early atherosclerosis as demonstrated by coronary angiography. *Atherosclerosis*, **26**, 151
2. Bulkley, B. H. and Roberts, W. C. (1975). The heart in systemic lupus erythematosus and the changes induced in it by corticosteroid therapy. *Am. J. Med.*, **58**, 243
3. Lindner, A., Charra, B., Sherrard, D. J. and Scribner, B. H. (1974). Accelerated atherosclerosis in prolonged maintenance hemodialysis. *N. Engl. J. Med.*, **290**, 697
4. Lowrie, E. G., Lazarus, J. M., Mocelin, A. J. *et al.* (1973). Survival of patients undergoing chronic hemodialysis and renal transplantation. *N. Engl. J. Med.*, **288**, 863
5. Kalbak, K. (1972). Incidence of arteriosclerosis in patients with rheumatoid arthritis receiving long-term corticosteroid therapy. *Ann. Rheum. Dis.*, **31**, 196
6. Etheridge, E. M. and Hoch-Ligeti, C. (1952). Lipid deposition in aortas in younger age groups following cortisone and adrenocorticotrophic hormone. *Am. J. Pathol.*, **28**, 315
7. Plotz, C. M., Knowlton, A. I. and Ragan, C. (1952). The natural history of Cushing's syndrome. *Am. J. Med.*, **13**, 597
8. Soffer, L. J., Iannaccone, A. and Gabrilove, J. L. (1961). Cushing's syndrome. A study of 50 patients. *Am. J. Med.*, **30**, 129
9. Jenkins, C. D. (1976). Recent evidence supporting psychologic and social risk factors for coronary disease. *N. Engl. J. Med.*, **294**, 1033
10. Rosenman, R. H., Brand, R. J., Jenkins, C. D., Friedman, M., Straus, R. and Wurm, M. (1975). Coronary heart disease in the Western Collaborative Group Study. Final follow-up experience of 8½ years. *J. Am. Med. Assoc.*, **233**, 872
11. Friedman, M., Byers, S. O. and Rosenman, R. H. (1972). Plasma ACTH and cortisol concentration of coronary-prone subjects. *Proc. Soc. Exp. Biol. Med.*, **140**, 681
12. Bagdade, J. D., Porte, D. and Bierman, E. L. (1970). Steroid-induced lipemia. *Arch. Intern. Med.*, **125**, 129
13. Kahn, C. R. (1980). Role of insulin receptors in insulin-resistant states. *Metabolism*, **29**, 455
14. Stamler, J., Pick, R. and Katz, L. N. (1954). Effects of cortisone, hydrocortisone and

corticotropin on lipemia, glycemia and atherogenesis in cholesterol-fed chicks. *Circulation*, **10**, 237

15. Friedman, M., Byers, S. and St George, S. (1964). Cortisone and experimental atherosclerosis. *Arch. Pathol.*, **77**, 142

16. Patterson, J. C. and Mitchell, C. A. (1951). Experimental coronary sclerosis. IV. The effect of cortisone on end-stage coronary sclerosis in chickens. *Arch. Pathol.*, **52**, 260

17. Malinow, M. R., Depaoli, R., Maruffo, C. A., Stevens, J., Szijan, I. and Kaplan, S. J. (1965). The effect of estradiol and hydrocortisone on atherosclerosis in cockerels. *J. Atheroscler. Res.*, **5**, 403

18. Rosenfeld, S., Marmorston, J., Sobel, H. and White, A. E. (1960). Enhancement of experimental atherosclerosis by ACTH in the dog. *Proc. Soc. Exp. Biol. Med.*, **103**, 83

19. Bagdade, J. D. and Stewart, M. (1977). Glucocorticoids and atherogenesis: serum factors stimulate the proliferation of human arterial smooth muscle cells. *Artery*, **3**, 360

20. Weinstein, R., Stemerman, M. B. and Maciag, T. (1981). Hormonal requirements for growth of arterial smooth muscle cells in vitro: an endocrine approach to atherosclerosis. *Science*, **212**, 818

21. Ronnemaa, T., Jarvelainen, H., Lehtonen, A. *et al.* (1980). Serum lipoprotein composition, hormones and the synthesis of glycosaminoglycans by human aortic smooth muscle cells. *Artery*, **8**, 323

22. Larjava, H., Saarni, H., Taami, M., Penttinen, R. and Ronnemaa, T. (1980). Cortisol decreases the synthesis of hyaluronic acid by human aortic smooth muscle cells in culture. *Atherosclerosis*, **35**, 135

23. Henze, K., Kudchodkar, B. J., Chait, A., Albers, J. J. and Bierman, E. L. (1981). The effect of hydrocortisone on cholesterol metabolism of cultured human skin fibroblasts. *Biochim. Biophys. Acta*, **666**, 199

19
Cyclic AMP

Adenosine-3′5′-cyclic monophosphate (cAMP) is a 'second messenger' in the action of a number of hormones[1,2]. Cyclic AMP mediates the glycogenolytic and lipolytic actions of glucagon and catecholamines. The actions of cAMP are, in general, opposite to the actions of insulin, but the role of cAMP in insulin action is not clear. The activity of platelets is also related to cAMP and increased platelet adhesiveness is associated with decreased cAMP[3].

As well as its metabolic activities, cAMP is involved in the regulation of cell division[4]. Cyclic AMP inhibits replication of a number of different cell lines in culture, and intracellular cAMP concentrations are inversely related to the rate of cell division. Malignant and transformed cells have low intracellular cAMP levels and growth control and morphological features can be restored towards normal by addition of dibutyryl cAMP to the culture medium. Most of the observations of the inhibitory effect of cAMP have been made on fibroblasts. In some other cell types, including hepatocytes, cAMP has the opposite action[5]. Guanosine cyclic 3′5′-monophosphate (cGMP) has opposite actions to cAMP.

As atherosclerosis is characterized by cellular proliferation and by abnormalities in the metabolism of arterial cells, cAMP may have a role in its pathogenesis and in the actions of hormones on the arterial wall. The evidence comes from experimental studies of the effects of cAMP on arterial tissue. The relation between circulating cAMP levels and atherosclerosis has not been studied, and in any case the significance of circulating cAMP is not clear.

Cyclic AMP has been identified in the arterial wall[6]. In cultured rabbit endothelial cells β-agonists increased cAMP concentrations while α-agonists increased cGMP levels[7]. Cyclic AMP production in cultured bovine aortic and pulmonary artery endothelial cells was increased by catecholamines (isoprenaline, adrenaline and noradrenaline) and prostaglandins (PGE_1, PGE_2 and $PGF_{2\alpha}$)[8]. Stimulation by isoprenaline was blocked by propranolol, a β-adrenoceptor blocking drug, but not by phentolamine, an α-adrenoceptor blocker. Other vasoactive agents including angiotensin I and II, bradykinin and serotonin had little effect on cAMP production. In cultured human umbilical venous endothelial cells the most potent stimulator of cAMP was prostacyclin (PGI_2) a labile prostaglandin which is a powerful vasodilator and the most potent inhibitor of human platelet aggregation yet described[9]. Stimulation of cAMP by PGI_2 was considerably greater than the stimulation observed with isoprenaline and the effect of PGI_2 was not affected by propranolol.

While it is clear that, in arterial tissue and isolated endothelial cells, cAMP is increased by vasoactive hormones, there have been no reports of the effects of other hormones on this process. There is also little information on the effects of either spontaneous or experimental atherosclerosis on cAMP levels in the arterial wall. However, in cholesterol-fed rabbits a low level of cAMP and high activity of cAMP phosphodiesterase was found in progressing atherosclerotic lesions and the reverse in regressing lesions[10]. Aortic segments from rabbits with experimental hypertension had decreased cAMP levels[11].

Dibutyryl cAMP inhibits DNA synthesis in cultured human endothelial cells[12,13] (Figure 19.1) and rat smooth muscle cells[13]. This effect was seen when the cells were grown in medium supplemented with whole serum or platelet poor serum but not when the cells were grown in the absence of serum. Dibutyryl cAMP also antagonized the stimulating effect of insulin on the proliferation of cultured primate aortic smooth muscle cells[14]. The

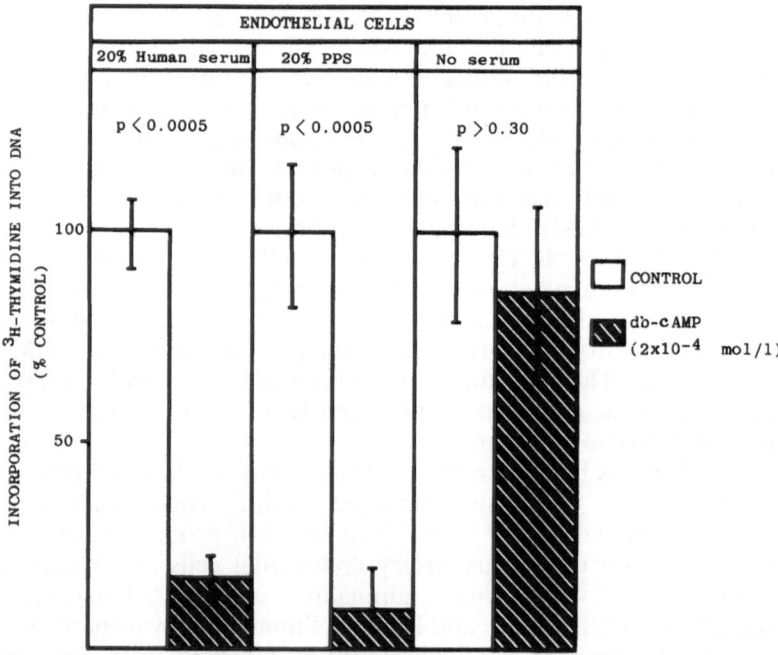

Figure 19.1 Effect of dibutyryl cAMP (2×10^{-4} mol/l) on DNA synthesis in cultured human umbilical venous endothelial cells, grown in medium supplemented with whole serum, platelet poor serum (PPS) or no serum[13]

pattern of response of endothelial and smooth muscle cells to cAMP was strikingly similar in view of the different responses of these cells to insulin and the platelet-derived growth factor[15].

Cyclic AMP also influences lipid metabolism in arterial tissue. In cultured rat aortic smooth muscle cells, dibutyryl cAMP inhibited sterol synthesis when the cells were grown in medium containing serum[16] and inhibited LDL binding to cultured human and rat arterial smooth muscle cells and human fibroblasts[17]. Cyclic AMP also inhibits sterol synthesis in the liver by influencing the activity of 3-hydroxy-3-methylglutaryl coenzyme A reductase, the rate-limiting enzyme in cholesterol synthesis[18,19].

There is no information on the effect of cAMP on connective tissue metabolism in the arterial wall. In chondrocytes dibutyryl cAMP enhances proteoglycan synthesis[20,21].

In conclusion, information on the relationship of cAMP to the biology of the arterial wall and to atherosclerosis is very limited. Arterial cAMP is regulated by vasoactive hormones and prostaglandins, and cAMP inhibits endothelial and smooth muscle cell replication and sterol binding and synthesis. The data are consistent with the other evidence that the artery is a hormone sensitive tissue.

References

1. Sutherland, E. W., Robison, G. A. and Butcher, R. W. (1968). Some aspects of the biological role of adenosine 3'5'-monophosphate (cyclic AMP). *Circulation*, **37**, 279
2. Sutherland, E. W. and Robison, G. A. (1969). The role of cyclic AMP in the control of carbohydrate metabolism. *Diabetes*, **18**, 797
3. Haslam, R. J., Davidson, M. M. L., Davies, T., Lynham, J. A. and McClenaghan, M. D. (1978). Regulation of platelet function by cyclic nucleotides. *Adv. Cyclic Nucl. Res.*, **9**, 533
4. Pastan, I. (1975). Regulation of cellular growth. *Adv. Metab. Disorders*, **8**, 7
5. McGowan, J. A., Strain, A. J. and Bucher, N. L. R. (1981). DNA synthesis in primary cultures of adult rat hepatocytes in a defined medium: effects of epidermal growth factor, insulin, glucagon and cyclic AMP. *J. Cell. Physiol.*, **108**, 353
6. Gilbert, C. H. and Galton, D. J. (1973). The presence of a hormone-sensitive cyclase system in the rat aorta and its relation to lipolysis. *Atherosclerosis*, **18**, 257
7. Buonassisi, V. and Venter, J. C. (1976). Hormone and neurotransmitter receptors in an established vascular endothelial cell line. *Proc. Natl. Acad. Sci. USA*, **73**, 1612
8. Makarski, J. S. (1981). Stimulation of cyclic AMP production by vasoactive agents in cultured bovine aortic and pulmonary artery endothelial cells. *In Vitro*, **17**, 450
9. Hopkins, N. K. and Gorman, R. R. (1981). Regulation of endothelial cell cyclic nucleotide metabolism by prostacyclin. *J. Clin. Invest.*, **67**, 540
10. Numano, F., Maezawa, H., Shimamoto, T. and Adachi, K. (1976). Changes of cyclic AMP and cyclic AMP phosphodiesterase in the progression and regression of experimental atherosclerosis. *Ann. NY Acad. Sci.*, **275**, 311
11. Tomera, J. F. and Harakal, C. (1980). Cyclic nucleotide changes in aortic segments derived from hypertensive rabbits. *Eur. J. Pharmacol.*, **68**, 505
12. Davison, P. M. and Karasek, M. A. (1981). Human dermal microvascular endothelial cells in vitro: effect of cyclic AMP on cellular morphology and proliferation rate. *J. Cell. Physiol.*, **106**, 253
13. Stout, R. W. (1982). Cyclic AMP: a potent inhibitor of DNA synthesis in cultured arterial endothelial and smooth muscle cells. *Diabetologia*, **22**, 51
14. Stout, R. W., Bierman, E. L. and Ross, R. (1975). Effect of insulin on the proliferation of cultured primate arterial smooth muscle cells. *Circulation*, **36**, 319

15. Taggart, H. and Stout, R. W. (1980). Control of DNA synthesis in cultured vascular endothelial and smooth muscle cells. *Atherosclerosis, 37,* 549
16. Stout, R. W. (1978). Relative insensitivity to glucagon of sterol synthesis in cultured rat aortic smooth muscle cells. Effect of dibutyryl cyclic AMP. *Diabetologia, 15,* 323
17. Stout, R. W. and Bierman, E. L. (1982). Dibutyryl cyclic AMP inhibits LDL binding in cultured fibroblasts and arterial smooth muscle cells. Atherosclerosis (in press)
18. Bricker, L. A. and Levey, G. S. (1972). Evidence for regulation of cholesterol and fatty acid synthesis in liver by cyclic adenosine 3'5'-monophosphate. *J. Biol. Chem., 247,* 4914
19. Beg, Z. H., Allmann, D. W. and Gibson, D. M. (1973). Modulation of 3-hydroxy-3-methylglutaryl coenzyme A reductase activity with cAMP and with protein fractions of rat liver cytosol. *Biochem. Biophys. Res. Commun., 54,* 1362
20. Miller, R. P., Husain, M. and Lohin, S. (1979). Long acting cAMP analogues enhance sulfate incorporation into matrix proteoglycans and suppress cell division of fetal rat chondrocytes in monolayer culture. *J. Cell. Physiol., 100,* 63
21. Speight, G., Handley, C. J. and Lowther, D. A. (1981). Effect of dibutyryl cyclic AMP on the sulphation of proteoglycans by chondrocytes. *Biochim. Biophys. Acta, 672,* 89

CONCLUSIONS

20
Conclusions

What is the relationship between hormone secretion and atherosclerosis? Is the relationship due to the direct effects of hormones on the arterial wall or is it mediated by changes in lipids, coagulation factors or other risk factors for atherosclerosis?

The strongest evidence linking hormones and atherosclerosis relates to diabetes and insulin. There is no doubt that hyperglycaemia increases the risk of cardiovascular disease. There is also recent evidence that high insulin levels have a predictive role in atherosclerosis. Mechanisms by which both high glucose and high insulin levels might promote the development of atherosclerosis have been described. Lipoprotein abnormalities, hypertension and abnormalities in platelet function may also have a role in this process.

For sex hormones, thyroid hormone, growth hormone and corticosteroids the evidence of a direct link with atherosclerosis is less strong, while for renin the evidence is weak. The nature of the association of the former hormones with cardiovascular disease suggests that it may be indirect. Evidence that the association is mediated entirely by changes in lipid and lipoprotein metabolism is not convincing. Changes in the sensitivity of arterial cells to risk factors is a possible mechanism but remains to be tested. It is notable that high plasma levels of all these hormones are associated with abnormal carbohydrate metabolism. This is a result of decreased sensitivity to the action of insulin, with hyperglycaemia and elevated insulin levels. The possibility that an association between sex hormones, thyroid hormone, growth hormone or corticosteroids and cardiovascular disease is mediated by changes in glucose and insulin is worthy of further study. Prospective studies of the relationship of glucose and insulin levels to atherosclerosis in these conditions are required. However, some of the hormone abnormalities are relatively rare so that the organization of such studies may be difficult.

Endocrinology has been a relatively neglected area of study in atherosclerosis research. In particular, there have been few studies of the direct effect of hormones on the arterial wall or on cultured arterial cells. It is likely that a greater research effort into hormone action in relation to cardiovascular disease will increase knowledge not only of endocrinology but also of atherosclerosis in general.

The importance of increasing knowledge of the development of atherosclerosis is the possibility that it may lead to prevention of cardiovascular disease. Prevention is probably an inappropriate concept. If atherosclerosis is basically an age-related process which may be accelerated by the addition of other factors, then delay rather than prevention should be the aim. Similar reservations apply to sentiments often expressed about the fact that cardiovascular disease is the commonest cause of death. Since the human lifespan is finite, everybody will eventually die, and some cause of death will be identified. With its close association with ageing, atherosclerosis and its complication of cardiovascular disease is likely to remain the commonest cause of death in older adults. It is premature death from atherosclerosis that is important and the identification of factors which accelerate atherosclerosis that is the challenge.

Of the factors that accelerate atherosclerosis, the male sex is the most potent. It seems more likely that the male sex promotes atherosclerosis than that the female sex prevents cardiovascular disease. However, it is not clear how the male sex promotes atherosclerosis or whether hormonal factors are involved. Since the higher incidence of atherosclerosis in males only occurs in areas of the world where the overall incidence of the disease is high it may be that the male sex in some way sensitizes the artery to other risk factors. Whatever the explanation, premature cardiovascular disease occurs in only a small proportion of men, and the general introduction of therapy directed at sex hormones cannot be justified.

Diabetes is another condition that is associated with premature atherosclerosis, in females as well as males. However, only about 2% of the population has diabetes and hence diabetes makes a relatively small contribution to the total burden of cardiovascular disease. None of the currently available methods of treating diabetes has been shown to prevent the development of cardiovascular disease in diabetics. However, even the best diabetic control is very different from normal carbohydrate metabolism and regulation of insulin secretion. Thus, the question as to whether 'cure' of diabetes will decrease the frequency of cardiovascular disease to that in non-diabetics cannot be answered at present. As with other risk factors, diabetes is too large and too crude a category and includes large numbers of people who will not develop premature cardiovascular disease. The next step will be to identify high-risk groups within those who have the currently defined risk factors.

The long-term adverse effects on the cardiovascular system of treatment such as oral hypoglycaemic drugs, oral contraceptives and oestrogens used in the treatment of prostatic carcinoma should induce caution in the long-term use of drugs or hormones in an attempt to delay atherosclerosis. It is still not widely appreciated that the concepts and requirements in preventing and treating chronic disease are quite different from those used in treating acute disease. On the evidence available at present there is no justification for prescribing hormones or hormone antagonists for the prevention of atherosclerosis.

Appendix

SI UNITS

Values of biochemical variables have been quoted in the way they appeared
in the original papers. Recent European publications have used SI units but
American and older European publications have used the older units. The
following is a brief conversion scale for the biochemical variables quoted in
this book.

	Older units	*SI units*
Cholesterol	200 mg/dl	5.18 mmol/l
	193.5 mg/dl	5 mmol/l
Creatinine	1 mg/dl	88.4 mmol/l
	1.13 mg/dl	100 mmol/l
Glucose	100 mg/dl	5.6 mmol/l
	90.1 mg/dl	5 mmol/l
Thyroxine	5 µg/dl	64.4 nmol/l
	7.78 µg/dl	100 nmol/l
Triiodothyronine	1 ng/ml	1.54 nmol/l
	1.3 ng/ml	2 nmol/l
Triglyceride	150 mg/dl	1.70 mmol/l
	177 mg/dl	2 mmol/l
Urea	50 mg/dl	8.3 mmol/l
	30.05 mg/dl	5 mmol/l

Index